The Menopause Relief Paradox

What Anger, Heat, Weight Gain, Cognitive Decline, and Immune Frailty Really is, and the 5 Easy Steps Any Woman Can Take to Reset the Mind-Body Connection

Maria Ian

Table of Contents

Foreword

This book began with a terrified young woman, desolate and alone in an impersonal, cold doctor's office. Not that the young woman had been informed that she has terminal cancer. That, at least, would have been a definite, clear answer to her many questions asked. For as much as her buzzing, fear-stricken brain could comprehend, she could have been suffering from cancer, leprosy, malaria, or from any of the host of other complex diseases. What else could she deduce from the evasive, confounding grumbling, echoing back at her from the distant yet stifling walls accompanied by the mechanical pushing onto a tablet? She had received as much in response to her answer to the question of her date of birth. The young woman concluded that her case certainly was the most unusual and distasteful. Muscle weakness, high blood pressure, laborious breathing, tingling in the hands and feet, chills, sweating, bloating, indigestion? Shaking legs? Panic and anxiety for no reason?

"E-hm," came the formal, ritualistic reaction. "This is normal … for your age." The young woman's world was thrown upside down. Strangely and irrationally, she suddenly, for a brief second, wished she had received that much expected diagnosis of cancer. At least that would have provided the needed hope that treatment, at least some action she could take, was at the end of this dismal tunnel. But … for her "age"?

Choking on dismay, the realization slowly but inexorably dawned on the young woman that she had been referred to as old, or at least as being older. Baffled speechless, the young woman felt that she had been placed by this eminent MD onto a slippery downwards slope, into a process placed outside of her control, at the end of which loomed death ugly, inevitable, and bigger than for that cancer patient that she now so dearly wished to be.

Nothing about that formal, ritualistic pronouncement made any conceivable sense. The young woman scrambled in her crammed mind for answers. How could any of this be? The only people she could denote as "old," on the spur of the moment in these accursed circumstances, had been in their upper nineties, whereas she herself was at only about one half of that number! The young woman confided in herself her secret aspiration, which was to reach her 60s, because the most amazing looking woman, sharp and shapely, she had ever known had been of that age! Certainly, so the young woman who was medically ignorant thought, there was something about that age that made a lady, a mystery she herself was yet to achieve? Her own mother, after all, had reached a certain peak at a time when she had been a decade beyond the young woman's present age! And why had the young woman encountered at least several older women who had never complained about the same ludicrous conditions, if such was just "normal, for her age"?

The young woman left the doctor's office alienated and perplexed. Certainly, it was something about that icy environment that now caused tremors in her legs, and her heart to flutter in her throat? Or ... maybe not? The young woman never returned to that horrific place.

Many of us, or the many women we know, have or will at a point in our lives experience one or several of the young woman's symptoms, commonly labeled as symptoms of Menopause.

Are all these symptoms related to menopause or cessation of menstrual periods?

The direct answer to this question is "NO" because many of these symptoms are not directly related to only cessation of periods or the female reproductive system, even though estrogen deficiency plays an important part in their evolution.

Take an example of increased anxiety in women in their 50s. Though cessation of periods can be one of the many possible explanations for this anxiety, there are many other more reasonable explanations for this: children leaving the home, retirement looming, exposure to psychological stress at a young age, exposure to domestic abuse, etc.

Similarly, vaginal dryness can occur due to the lack of or much decreased sexual activity (a more reasonable explanation rather than menopause) Thus, physical, and psychological manifestations of women who experience menopause should not always be attributed to that stage in a woman's life. To better understand this, we have to consider these symptoms collectively as the human body works as a single unit instead of separate and independent systems.

The human body as a single unit

Though it contains different systems and organs, the human body works as a single unit. All these organs and systems work in combination to make the body work.

It includes not only anatomical structures of our body but also emotions and behaviors. For example, if you have severe pain in the right foot, is it possible to be excited and happy even if you heard the best of news? The answer would be No.

Why? Because our body is overall connected and working together. That also explains the phenomenon of death when all the organs are placed in their anatomical locations, but the body stops functioning as a whole. If the systems worked separately without their wholeness, some systems might continue working for years, even after death.

The Western Medical literature explains this whole-body concept in instances. According to Western Medicine, severe and persistent mental stress, for example, can lead to gastric ulcers and increased glucose levels (Both are organic manifestations of psychological issues).

Similarly, Traditional Chinese Medicine (TCM) endorses the concept of the human body as one integrated whole created to work together in harmony. According to the TCM practitioners, the specific root cause of menopause symptoms is not the female reproductive tract or cessation of ovulation. Multiple organs, such as the kidney, liver, heart, spleen, etc., are studied to play a role in these symptoms.

Explanation of Menopause symptoms under this concept:

Considering the human body as one whole being, it is not justifiable to attribute all the so-called menopausal symptoms as manifestations of anovulation occurring in the female reproductive tract.

Exploring different explanations of these symptoms reveals that they are so variable that they can only be explained if you consider the human body working together, not a collection of organs or systems. To explain it further, let's have a brief review of some of the manifestations under this concept,

- Physiologic stressors that a woman faces during adolescence, adulthood, and middle age accumulate in different body parts. As a result, bones get brittle and weak from this stress; anxiety attacks become more prevalent; concentration levels become low; and sleep disturbances in the 50s. A woman's body gets osteoporosis, hot flashes, memory disturbances, and insomnia, respectively, occurring in different parts of the body. At the same time, the origin of these symptoms is the same, i.e., physiologic stressors that a woman experienced during her earlier life.

- Nutritional deficiencies such as mineral loss, vitamin deficiencies, and low calcium levels often attributed to menopause are only reflections of gastrointestinal disturbances and low intake during middle age. Having too many gastrointestinal disturbances, such as chronic diarrhea, lactose intolerance, malabsorption syndromes, etc., can lead to long-term nutritional deficiencies.

- Explanation of menopause symptoms should also include the cellular level concept rather than only focusing on the organ or system level. Mitochondrial dysfunction is the perfect example of that. Although mitochondria are a small organelle located within a cell, their dysfunction can lead to failure of or decreased antioxidant and anti-inflammatory activities of the body at any age, and certainly if left uncared for prolonged periods. Thus, the symptoms of menopause are better explained if we take the human body as one whole entity containing different systems and organs that influence each other. This whole entity contains billions of cells containing many organelles. If even one type of organelles is not functioning properly, the manifestations can become apparent in the body.

It is not ending here.

Keeping in view the facts mentioned above, the focus in the next chapters will include an explanation of menopause symptoms, their effects on our body, possible management options, including the use of our body's energy to alleviate these symptoms, and steps that you can take from a younger age to prevent yourselves from these symptoms at a later age.

Keep in mind as you read this book:

As you read this book, keep in mind that none of the symptoms discussed happen on their own. Our bodies are extraordinarily complex, and what happens in one place, inevitably affects another place, even if we do not know what happened in the first place at all.

That is to say that we cannot treat symptoms in isolation. But as many of us have experienced, that is what the majority of medical practitioners today has as their focus, for the sake of time expediency, prescriptions of medications, short sighted and narrow-minded financial gain.

Be encouraged to ask your medical practitioner about the interrelatedness of your symptoms. Demand specific and detailed answers. If he or she is dismissive or the answer is unsatisfactory, do not be intimidated, embarrassed, or afraid to find another practitioner who is willing to help. Do so immediately, not once symptoms have become worse, or you have gone through all rational justifications.

Remember, it is your health. Once your health is gone, it is either gone, or extremely difficult to recuperate. That progression affects each and every human. In the present moment, only very few of us think that they will ever suffer that affliction. But the reasons to care are abundant. Our bodies have been amazingly designed to heal themselves. You owe it to yourself to find out.

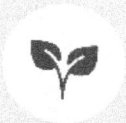

WANT A DEEP DIVE INTO WHAT MAKES OUR BODIES TICK?

FOR FREE PREVIEWS OF UPCOMING PUBLICATIONS, HEALTH & WELLNESS TIPS, AND FREE RECIPIES

JOIN MY MAILING LIST, EMAIL 'SUBSCRIBE ME' AND WHITELIST

MARIAIANAUTHOR@GMAIL.COM

I DON'T SELL OR GIVE OUT YOUR EMAIL ADDRESS EVER

Introduction:

Why Is This Happening to Me?

Life is supposed to be a wild ride, full of ups and downs, twists, and turns. We cannot help but notice a larger purpose, a mysterious yet very real design that can help guide us through it all. We rarely stop to think how our own bodies go through something very similar. Nature, in its infinite wisdom, by means of hundreds of thousands of years of evolution, has made sure of it.

Everything changes, even our planet goes through cycles, its path around the sun ebbs and flows too slowly for any living creature to notice. The devil is in the details, and only very few among us stop to listen. Fresh green leaves sprout when least expected, no matter how cold or dry the previous season was. Against all odds, life has proven to be persistent, and ungovernable at its essence. Continents drift, climate changes, species evolve, have their time in the sun, and eventually become extinct. The only constant in nature, is change.

Change is scary, but also exiting, and necessary, as things that do not evolve tend to stagnate. Some of us might remember the harsh pain throbbing in our hips and in our legs when, for the first time as toddlers, we had to obey nature's call to get up, stand tall, and start to walk. We all would have preferred to stay children but think of all the things you would have missed, becoming independent, finding your calling, falling in love, and having children of your own. Looking back, the catalyst behind these extraordinary experiences, the reason for coming into this world and taking one's first step, is one big mystery.

Of course, when you're a kid, going through puberty, you don't see it that way. Your body start to change, you feel weird, sometimes gross, sometimes angry, or emotional for no reason. It is confusing and scary, especially if you don't have someone to guide you through.

But nature knows what it's doing, our bodies are ultimately perfect in their own ways. Eventually, once we're on the other side, it all makes sense. Our body had to change, just like the caterpillar, because it has to prepare for what comes next.

The same can be said about menopause. But if all these changes are a natural part of life, why do we at times feel like there's something really wrong happening to us? Why do we dread change, instead of celebrating that our body is preparing for what's next? Because some symptoms really suck, and because there are things that throw our body out of balance, making it worse than it needs to be.

Don't panic! Last time nature caught us by surprise, this time we are ready. With age comes wisdom, we are more mature, and now we are ready to get in front of mother nature and welcome her with open arms, her vices, quirks, as well as joys included. Hopeful, by the end of this book, we may have received at least some knowledge on how we can benefit from braving the unknown.

Menopause, as we all know, is the moment in a woman's life when menstruation stops permanently. But that is not all. So much more is going on besides this one symptom that medical professionals utilize to define when menopause has occurred.

There are other symptoms, the most typical are hot flashes, a sudden wave of heat, that can last between thirty seconds to ten minutes, even though they feel like they last forever. With hot flashes, come other symptoms, including trouble sleeping, and mood changes, which in all honesty, is understandable if you ever experienced the hot flashes. This period of transition can go on for several years, a not insignificant amount of time to be uncomfortable and in distress.

Menopause typically comes around between the 47th and 54th birthdays, even though there are factors that can cause a woman to go into early menopause, such as heavy smoking or having an untreated celiac disease. Some medical procedures, such as chemotherapy or certain types of surgery that remove the uterus or the ovaries, can also bring on early menopause.

The first thing to understand about menopause, is that difficult as it can be, it is not a disease or disorder. It is not meant to be frowned upon in a doctor's office, even though, it can aggravate other underlying conditions that can potentially warrant seeking medical care.

Menopause is a natural change, and if we're healthy, mindful, and informed, there is no reason to be scared. The main cause for these changes is the depletion of eggs in the ovaries. A woman is born with a finite number of oocytes, these are the cells that each month mature into an egg as part of the menstrual cycle. This means that every woman, since before they're born, already have all the eggs they will use throughout the rest of their life. And anything in nature that has a beginning definitely will have an end.

The Three Stages of Menopause

Menopause doesn't happen all at once, and it doesn't happen the same for everyone, for some women, menstruation can just suddenly stop without symptoms, others might have a harder time. This all depends on many factors, and just because you have a harder or easier time than others, doesn't mean you're not healthy.

For its study, menopause it is divided in three stages, the first of which is called perimenopause. The literal meaning of the term is "approaching menopause" and it starts years before menstruation stops. This is a transition period, and because symptoms start mildly, it is difficult to know when you have entered perimenopause, as is the case with pretty much every stage of menopause, the boundaries tend to blur. It can last from four to eight years, during which women are still fertile, and is to significant extent related to a woman's hormones.

There are two main female sex hormones, estrogen, and progesterone. Estrogen is mostly produced in the ovaries, and plays the main role in reproduction, sex, and development. It plays an important role during pregnancy and is responsible for puberty, menstruation, and menopause. It also has a vital role in regulating and protecting the brain, cardiovascular system, hair, skin, urinary tract, and musculoskeletal system.

Progesterone is produced by the ovaries after ovulation, its job is to make the lining of the uterus ready to receive a fertilized egg, to support it during pregnancy, and to tell the ovaries to stop producing estrogen after ovulation.

There are other sex hormones, like estradiol, which is responsible for the development of sexual characteristics during puberty, like breasts and widening of the hips. It also has significant effects in other tissues, like bone, fat, skin, liver, and the brain. Women also produce small amounts of testosterone, as it is an essential hormone for bone and muscle strength, as well as sex drive.

During a normal menstrual cycle, the ovaries, still brimming with oocytes, produce a cocktail of hormones, like estrogen, estradiol, progesterone, even some testosterone. During perimenopause, the levels of these hormones start rising and falling unevenly, causing the cycles to become irregular.

The second stage is just called menopause, after oocytes finally run out, menstruation stops, after 12 consecutive months without it, you're officially in menopause. During the last couple of years before officially reaching menopause, changes in hormone levels start causing physical symptoms. There are many other aspects of our bodies, that we tend not to think about much. We take our health for granted and hit the snooze button, sometimes for as long as a decade or two. It's during this stage, that our lack of vigilance can come back to haunt us.

Who remembers when, as a kid, we became addicted to marshmallow fluff, maybe we used sugary treats as comfort food in moments of sadness, or when we were grossed out by veggies? Back then, a tummy ache meant to take just another Pepto-Bismol, and we'd bounce right back. But now, like a broken-down car left at the side of the road because another part of us can afford to rush off and buy a new one, it won't be so easy to shrug off physical symptoms. And before we know it, our woes pile up more numerous than the stars in the sky.

Finally, it's time to pay the piper. The withdrawal from a lifetime supply of hormones now meets a body depleted of strength, and as our bodies can no longer keep up, we are left limping on one leg.

The symptoms most women experience at this stage include: vasomotor symptoms (hot flashes), night sweats, difficulty sleeping, mood swings, vaginal dryness, loss of muscle mass, a leaching of calcium in the bones, and an increase in body fat. Also, menopausal women are more likely to develop neurodegenerative diseases, like Alzheimer's; cardiovascular disease, like arteriosclerosis; and other chronic and degenerative diseases, such as osteoporosis.

It is also associated with higher likelihood of depression, anxiety, and irritability, symptoms that we usually only associate with our mental state.

Post menopause is the final stage, post meaning "after". If it's been more than a year since your last period, congratulations, you're done with menopause, although technically, you will be in post menopause for the rest of your life. Since periods are erratic during the previous stage, it is difficult to determine when exactly Aunt Flo visited last, that is why you have to wait a full year, before you can legally declare her dead.

Even after entering post menopause, some symptoms may linger on, interacting in different ways with the typical signs of aging. But as our bodies adjust to the new reality, symptoms should diminish over time. Symptoms should be replaced by strengths, such as an expanded awareness or consciousness, new intellectual interests, creative pursuits, that we previously may not have known we possessed. If this doesn't happen, it might be a sign of a more dangerous underlying condition.

When you get down to the nitty-gritty, menopause symptoms are caused by hormonal imbalances, that with nothing to balance them out, can result in an unregulated bush fire. In our bodies, like in nature, everything is connected, and everything happens for a reason. We are a complex system, full of interaction, and what happens to one part, like the ovaries, affects the whole organism. Hormone imbalance left at the center of it, will not benefit nature with the wisdom that she deserves.

Taken in isolation and looked with the cold dispassionate objectivity of a sterile lab setting, hormones regulate a lot more than just the menstrual cycle. Hormones are chemical messengers, they travel in your bloodstream, from one tissue to another one, regulating various processes, working slowly over time.

They control growth, our circadian rhythm, which is our internal clock that controls our wake-sleep cycle; they regulate our mood, appetite, immune response, and our metabolism. They even influence how we form long term memories and our cognition, plus, a lot of other very important bodily functions, that will be discussed in detail over the coming chapters.

Overproduction of hormones is also called hyperfunction or hypersecretion, while underproduction of hormones is referred to as hypofunction or hyposecretion. Hyper or hypo production can happen for several reasons, it can be due to a genetic disorder, sometimes a tumor can affect a gland, causing it to produce abnormal quantities of a hormone.

Under normal circumstances, hormones are regulated by what's called a homeostatic negative feedback control system. This is a complicated way of saying that when the body senses an overproduction of hormones, it slows down the rate at which they're being pumped out, until the blood hormone levels even out.

This is not triggered by the actual number of hormones present in your system, but rather by the "effect" of that hormone. Think about it as someone at a party, that instead of counting how many drinks they have, they stop drinking when they feel tipsy.

So, for most of your adult life, your body is chugging along producing estrogen, estradiol, and progesterone. This last one tells your ovaries that it's time to prepare a beautiful egg. So, the oocyte becomes an egg, you ovulate, and it goes forth into the world, hopefully to become a baby. Then your body says, — "thanks ovaries, see you next month", and stops producing progesterone, until it's needed again.

But, since there's a limited number of eggs, they eventually run out, but your body doesn't know that. So, it keeps pushing the progesterone button, sending the message to ovulate over and over, but the ovaries can't do anything about it. This causes, the hormone levels to spike. And this is the start of a cascading effect that can get out of control pretty quick, since sex hormones control a lot of other things in your body. Soon things start going crazy.

Progesterone doesn't work alone, like a team of superheroes, they have sidekicks, that join in and gang up on you. For example, estrogen amplifies the physiological effects of progesterone, this creates a chain of events that end up affecting the delicate balance in your body. To give you an idea, here is a brief, and not at all comprehensive list of other things that progesterone affects:

- Skin health: Our skin is protected by a protein called collagen, decreased levels of progesterone result in loss of collagen, which results in loss of elasticity, thinner skin, and wrinkling.

- Neurotransmitters: Sex hormones regulate the function of serotonin receptors, the neurotransmitters that are released by our brain's reward system, basically what lets you enjoy things. It also helps regulate mood; this is why so many women experience depression.

- Core temperature: Through several mechanisms, which we will discuss in chapter one, our core body temperature is regulated by several mechanisms which are mediated by hormones. When these go, you get hot flashes.

- Water retention: Progesterone plays an important balance in sodium levels. When it starts to fail, it causes water retention, making you feel bloated.

- Our immune system is regulated by hormones, which in turn have a significant effect on inflammation, and our gut health.

- Our metabolism and energy balance are maintained and controlled by hormones, through several mechanisms that affect us at the cellular level.

- Estrogen is an antioxidant, that plays a vital role in preventing oxidative stress, a very important concept we will be discussing.

The list is long, but it doesn't end there, because once you start messing with things like your sleep cycle, or your immune system, it can cause a chain reaction that gets out of hand very quickly.

It all sounds scary, and sometimes all these things coming at you at the same time can make you feel like you have no say in the matter, but it is not so. There is good reason to stay positive because nature has got your back. Understanding the changes in our body, and the underlying processes behind the symptoms, is the best way to take back control. So here are five of the main interactions that cause most of the symptoms we experience during menopause, but also five easy steps to see you through it.

Chapter 1:

Physiological Stressors: They Will Kill You Unless You Stop Them Now

The Neuroendocrinology of Stress

Think of the humble honeybee. A hive is composed of millions of individuals, each carrying out a specific job, in perfect coordination, maintaining an equilibrium and harmony that help propagate life and make our world more beautiful. At the core of every beehive, there is one individual that is unique among all the others, the queen bee.

The queen is the mother of all other bees. Through a complex system of chemical messaging, she runs the hive like a well-tuned piece of machinery. But as the queen ages, and passes her reproductive age, a new queen is born to replace her. The new queen will soon fly away and produce her own offspring, but before this happens, the worker bees, swarm around the previous queen in a tight, smothering embrace.

This is called balling, and in a certain poetic way is a formidable catastrophe. The heat generated by this congregation, ends up suffocating the queen mother, and she ends her days surrounded by all her children. As anyone who's been through menopause can attest, hot flashes can make you feel like you are burning to death. Also, at this stage in life, we're usually also dealing with situations in our families, work, health problems and many other situations, that can make us feel like we're being swarmed and smothered.

A lot more is going on in your body than just heat. Situations in life cause us mental and physical stress, which interacts and compounds the natural symptoms of our transition. Both kinds of stress are detrimental to our health, and should be addressed immediately, however the cause for physiological stress can be harder to pinpoint. That physiological stress is more relevant than psychological is fascinating and will strike many readers as unusual and interesting, particularly since we will be emphasizing mindfulness.

Of course, none of this is meant to be. Nature made us perfect. Homeostasis is the natural tendency of our bodies towards a state of equilibrium. Whenever any stimuli, real or perceived, from within or without, threatens this fragile balance, that is what we call physiological stress. For brevity's sake, we'll just call it stress, but keep in mind that unless otherwise specified, I mean physiological, not psychological stress.

To maintain this balance, nature in its wisdom, has equipped us with a sophisticated system that redirects energy according to the body's needs. It is called the stress system. Its job is to adjust and react to stimuli that upset this balance, also known as stressors. A bit of stress is beneficial. Stress helps motivate us and can make us stronger. You can't create diamonds without pressure, and trees need wind to grow strong. But when the stressor becomes excessive or prolonged, or when other circumstances may cause it to surpass our system's ability to adapt, then we're in trouble.

When stressors persist over a long time, they can compromise mental and physical health, even life expectancy. In those cases, our nervous and endocrine systems team up to help the body adapt and overcome the stressor.

The endocrine system's job is to be the messenger between different organs and other systems in your body. It does this by using several internal glands, located throughout or body, to create and release several hormones directly into the circulatory system. The endocrine system works together with your nervous system, all the different nerves that relay information from the body to your brain.

The endocrine system is in charge of preparing the complex cocktails of hormones that our body uses to regulate its functions. One of the endocrine system's tools is what is called a "flight or fight" response. We usually arrive to this state when scared or angry. It is our body's way to prepare us for bad things to go down.

When our brain detects a stressor, it tells our endocrine system to start pumping us full of hormones. The main one is adrenaline because it has the most important role in this reaction. You are probably familiar with this one. Adrenaline is secreted whenever we do anything exiting or scary, it gives you butterflies in your stomach. Its job is to make you more alert and focused. Adrenaline does this by increasing blood flow to your muscles, so you're ready to spring into action. This blood is taken from parts of your body that are less essential in a danger situation, your face, and your digestive system. This is why when you see a ghost, you turn pale, and feel a pit in your stomach.

Adrenaline also raises your hearth rate, because in a fight you need extra oxygen, so you feel your heart pounding in your chest and your ears. It dilates your bronchi, the tubes that move air into your lungs, so you can get more air; and adrenaline relaxes the bladder walls, because crying in a roller coaster is not humiliating enough, you also have to wet your pants.

Cortisol is another hormone made in your adrenal glands. Cortisol is released as a response to stress. Normally, cortisol is produced in lower quantities, and it helps regulate our sleep-wake cycle and our immune system. Cortisol also participates in controlling our blood sugar by counteracting insulin, playing an important role in our metabolism.

When we are under stress for a prolonged length of time, our bodies keep producing cortisol in response. After a while, it floods our bloodstream, and starts interfering with things like bone formation, contributing to the loss of density in our bones, which can eventually cause chronic pathologies, like osteoporosis. Cortisol messes with the balance of electrolytes, making us to retain sodium and water and causing bloating; it also stimulates the secretion of stomach acids, which is why people with high stress jobs suffer from heartburn.

Cortisol and adrenaline work together to create memories of short-term emotional events, having a part in the mechanism of trauma and PTSD. However, long exposure to elevated cortisol levels can eventually damage the hippocampus, the part of our brain in charge of long-term memory and learning, that is also involved in the production of neurotransmitters that regulate our mood.

There are many situations that can act as long-term stressors. Chronic pain, emotional trauma, a dangerous or unhealthy environment and toxins all can cause us to be in a prolong state of fight or flight. One situation that commonly is at the top of the list of stressors in menopausal women are hot flashes.

Vasomotor Symptoms

This is the fancy science name for hot flashes. Vasomotor symptoms or VMS are the hallmark symptom of menopause, as a majority of women will experience hot flashes at some point in their life. Symptoms often start during the perimenopausal period and can last throughout menopause and even beyond the postmenopausal phase.

Hot flashes vary in intensity, not only from person to person, but within individual women. The mild ones manifest as a brief warming sensation, while the more intense ones feel are a sudden and extreme heat that spreads over the body and face.

They are accompanied by intense transpiration, which is referred to as "night sweats", but can also occur during the day. Other symptoms that can accompany hot flashes include pressure in the head or chest, anxiety, nausea, changes in heart rate and breathing. They can also be a major factor in sleep disturbances, anxiety, and depression.

These comorbidities could be a serious issue, because, aside from being uncomfortable, there is evidence that VMS represents a chronic stress condition with important health implications, so let's unpack how VMS work.

We mentioned how our bodies maintain an internal equilibrium called homeostasis, this includes maintaining a constant temperature. Humans like all other mammals are endotherms. We have the ability to regulate our body temperature, through our metabolism, by using stored energy to heat up; unlike for example reptiles, which are ectotherms, meaning they need to bask in the sun to heat, and have a very slow metabolism.

When this mammalian superpower to raise and lower our body temperature is functioning normally, we maintain a core body temperature of 98,6 °F (37 °C). This is the ideal temperature for our organs to function, and we maintain it regardless of the temperature outside our body (within reason).

The physiological control of our body's core temperature takes place primarily in a part of our brain called the hypothalamus, which works as the body's thermostat. Through nerve cells called thermoreceptors, the hypothalamus receives signals from key temperature sensors throughout our body, telling it that is either too hot or too cold.

If it is too cold, and our core body temperature drops below the optimal range, our brain signals our body to turn up the heat. The hypothalamus sends a signal through nerves from the sympathetic nervous system. This is the part of our nervous system that controls the fight or flight response, and it gives the signal for blood to flow away from our skin, sending it instead to the internal organs to keep them warm. Then, our muscles start to contract, generating heat by shivering, and causing our hairs to stand on end, giving us goosebumps.

When instead our body temperature is too high, the same system makes blood flow to the skin, where it is closer to the outside of the body. Then it tells our skin to start producing sweat, which cools down our skin and the blood beneath as it evaporates. All this signaling back and forth between the sympathetic nervous system, the hypothalamus, our skin, organs, and blood vessels, is regulated by hormones.

During perimenopause, estrogen and estradiol levels begin to fluctuate. It is this period of unpredictable swings in hormone levels that causes directly or indirectly most symptoms during menopause, including VMS. The exact mechanism behind it is still being debated in the scientific community, but there are three likely hypotheses.

The first and most prominent is that the hormonal mayhem experienced during menopause alters the thresholds for acceptable body temperature. Even small changes in our core body temperature can trigger a thermoregulatory response. Basically, the hypothalamus gets confused and raises the threshold at which it tells your body it's too cold and lowers the one at which it tells it's too hot.

In support of this theory, studies have shown that for some women, hot flashes were preceded by an almost insignificant increase in core body temperature that would have been tolerated under normal circumstances, but that triggered an exaggerated response.

A second hypothesis proposes that VMS is the consequence of a change in the responsiveness in peripheral vasculature. Normally, our skin reacts to changes in temperature by increasing or diminishing blood flow, it does this by dilating or contracting the tiny capillaries and small veins near the surface of the skin. Since estrogen and progesterone both influence skin blood flow control, changes in these hormone levels may cause blood vessels to react more slowly to changes in temperature, causing an exaggerated response.

Also, low levels of estradiol affect the threshold for dilation of blood vessels. This is similar to theory number one, except here, it is the blood vessels who are to blame for changing the threshold for thermoregulation not the brain.

The third hypothesis states that during a premenopausal woman's life, hormonal levels go through a monthly cycle. Estrogen levels start to rise from the first day of menses to tell the ovaries to prepare to release the egg, then drop precipitously after ovulation. This is followed by a second rise in estrogen around day fourteen of the cycle, after which estrogen levels start decreasing until it is time to begin the cycle again.

The brain is used to dealing with these regular monthly changes. But when these fluctuations become unpredictable, parts of the brain that are highly hormone responsive, like the hypothalamus, are unable to adapt fast enough, so they're having delayed reactions to hormone levels that fluctuate faster than they can adapt.

The hypothalamus is the region of the brain in charge of integrating all the thermal information from the body and controlling the thermoregulatory response. Decreasing hormone levels leads to changes in the balance of neurotransmitters that manage this part of the brain, causing the regulatory response to be compromised.

So which theory is it? Hard to say, there is good evidence for each one, and since they're not mutually exclusive, it's probably a combination of all three. The unpredictability of hormone levels is a significant factor in each.

There is evidence that estradiol is the main hormone responsible for hot flashes, and hormone replacement therapy has shown effectiveness in alleviating these symptoms. However, for the majority of women, the symptoms come back after stopping taking hormones, which suggests that over time the brain needs to adapt to different neurochemical levels, by adjusting its reactions to match the new levels. How long that adaptation period takes varies from one individual to another.

One of the bigger risks associated with VMS is that they may play a causal role in other symptoms. The most common is sleep deprivation, as hot flashes constantly interrupt sleep, leading to other cognitive issues.

Also, there is evidence that severe VMS can cause premature aging in cells, leading to alterations in gene expression that can potentially compromise cell function. This is a consequence of persistent stress causing oxidative stress, which results in accumulated damage to DNA over the years. Our cells are equipped to repair this molecular wear and tear, but when external factors accelerate DNA damage, it can have serious consequences.

For example, oxidative stress can cause epigenetic alterations of the immune system. Epigenetic alterations occur when cells don't properly control gene activity. These alterations can suppress the activation of immune cells, causing inflammation and an attenuated immune response, leaving us vulnerable to pathogens. We will discuss the role of oxidative stress, inflammation, and the immune system in later chapters. For now, let's focus on the cascading effect of vasomotor symptoms.

Sleep Disturbances: The "Domino Effect"

We all need our beauty sleep. The quality and quantity of our rest directly affects our nervous system. If we don't get our 7-8 hours, we start getting cranky, complex tasks become difficult, and it's common to have headaches, even hallucinations. Over longer periods of time, lack of sleep can seriously impact our cognitive abilities.

There are several medical conditions that have detrimental effects on the quality of sleep. However, there is a very well-studied relationship between VMS, depressive symptoms, and sleep disturbances. This relationship is explained through the "domino effect". It states that night sweats caused by VMS may be the cause of sleep disturbances that, in turn, correlate with depressive symptoms.

Night sweats make it impossible to sleep. You are awakened by a pounding heart, or the sudden sensation of being in a furnace. Women with VMS that reported having a depressive disorder also reported difficulty in falling sleep, reduced quality, and overall duration of sleep. Even if depression pulls you into sleep, VMS can cause you to suddenly become alert. If you are the smart type that thinks right now, I should be optimizing my vascular health and my emotional well-being, then yes, you are on the right track, with no return ticket allowed!

To put it simply, hot flashes make it hard to fall asleep, and can cause interruptions in the sleep cycle. Over a period of time, this leads to more serious health problems, depression, and irritability.

Depressive Symptoms

Everyone feels sad sometimes, maybe you've had a bad day or got some bad news, perhaps someone close passed away. These feelings are normal as they are part of the human experience. You can't appreciate the good times without the bad. Depression however is a whole different animal.

Depression is more than occasionally feeling blue. Depression is a mood disorder, a mental health condition that affects our emotional state. Usually, it involves a chemical imbalance that changes the way you feel, think, and handle daily activities, such as sleeping, eating, or working. There are many situations that can cause a bout with depression, called a major depressive disorder, like prolonged stress, trauma, PTSD, or a genetic predisposition.

According to the Diagnostic and Statistical Manual of Mental Disorders, Fifth Edition, or DSM-5, to be diagnosed with a major depressive disorder, it requires suffering of at least five of the following symptoms for at least two weeks:

- Feelings of sadness, anxiety, or "emptiness", persisting over a prolonged period

- Irritability

- Feelings of guilt, worthlessness, hopelessness or pessimism, or helplessness

- Loss of interest in hobbies or activities previously enjoyed

- Low energy or persistent fatigue

- Sluggishness, apathy, moving or talking more slowly

- Restlessness, having trouble sitting still

- Difficulty concentrating, remembering things, and making decisions

- Problems sleeping, getting up in the morning, or oversleeping

- Increased appetite or sudden weight changes

- Idealization of death or suicide

- Aches, pains, headaches, cramps, or digestive problems with no apparent reason, or that won't go away with treatment

If you're suffering from one or more of these symptoms, please put down this book and seek help. Depression is no joke, but it can be overcome. There are several free resources and help available[1]. And if you or someone else you know is having a psychiatric emergency, please call 911.

There is a new appreciation of perimenopause and the early postmenopausal years as being associated with an increased risk of depression. However, this is a complicated issue. Many factors that can complicate and overlap with menopause symptoms and result in a depressive episode that was developing or was already there.

Numerous studies have found that depressive symptoms were significantly more prevalent in perimenopausal versus premenopausal women, as 45% to 68% of perimenopausal women reported elevated depressive symptoms compared with 28% to 31% of premenopausal women (Maki et al., 2019). These percentages were constant, even in women with no previous history of depression, but especially in those who had experienced adverse life events or vasomotor symptoms during perimenopause.

Even if there is no direct physiological link between menopause and depression, during this period women often experience elevated psychological distress. This can be related to factors like taking care of aging parents, while still taking care of children, work, and relationships.

Add to this stressors like the sleep disturbances caused by vasomotor symptoms, and you just might have a recipe for a perfect storm. Women suffering from hot flashes, that reported reduced quality and

---

[1] Please go to https://nndc.org/resource-links/ for more information.

quantity of sleep, are more likely to develop a major depressive disorder. Which is understandable, since years of being tired all the time, waking up in the middle of the night in a pool of sweat, and feeling like you're on fire can't be great for your mental health.

Importantly, depression and anxiety have been linked to oxidative stress. Oxidative stress is when the antioxidants that are meant to protect the cells from free radicals are outmatched by free radicals. As free radicals are formed, oxygen atoms with an unpaired electron that are highly reactive and unstable oxidize DNA, causing cellular damage. Free radicals are a byproduct of our metabolism, so the greater the energy requirements of an organ, the greater is the production of Reactive Oxygen Species (ROS), another name for free radicals.

The brain is a particular energy demanding organ since neurons have very high metabolisms and lower endogenous levels of antioxidants compared to other cells. This higher oxidative stress in turn causes inflammation, and both oxidative and inflammatory processes are interconnected with depression.

Sleep deprivation is also a factor that increases the oxidative stress. When we are awake, (i.e., being awake simmering in a pool of sweat), our brains are in a heightened state of alertness, requiring more energy and oxygenation. The brain metabolism remains high and consequently, there is a higher rate of formation of ROS. During sleep, neurological activity is lower, and the levels of several hormones rise, like melatonin and human growth hormone (HGH), that act as antioxidants, protecting the brain from oxidation.

Oxidative stress can impair the function of neurotransmitters like serotonin and dopamine in our brains. Over time, this imbalance can increase the risk of mental disorders, like major depressive disorder. It also leads to a dysregulation of circadian rhythms, which further aggravates sleeping disturbances, creating a feedback loop that can easily spiral out of control.

The usual treatment for depression consists of antidepressants and cognitive-behavioral therapy (CBT). The latter is a kind of psychotherapy that helps patients identify and get rid of negative thoughts about themselves, and their past, present, and future situations, that promote depression. Clinical trials show that CBT also improves depressive symptoms related to menopause.

Various randomized studies in older women with major depressive disorder suggest that estrogen therapy may augment the response to SSRIs, selective serotonin reuptake inhibitors, one common type of antidepressant. They also demonstrated a positive effect on VMS severity, sleep disturbances, anxiety, and pain in perimenopausal and postmenopausal women.

Other interesting results show that after 12 months of receiving estradiol as part of hormone therapy, women were significantly less likely to develop depression, compared with women receiving placebo. These same studies showed greater benefits for women that in the six months prior experienced stressful life events, suggesting that women in early perimenopausal stage may benefit more than women in later stages of menopause.

Even after suspending hormone treatment, the antidepressant effects of estradiol remained, despite the re-emergence of VMS and night sweats. So even if HRT can help with depression, it is not a permanent fix as many women complained about unwelcomed side effect, and of other symptoms returning after suspending treatment.

Hopefully, some information in this book will give readers hope, in that by taking care in time of their vascular health, emotional well-being, and other recommendations to be discussed, they can gain the upper hand. Do not wait for symptoms to develop, or to reach any specific age, before being pro-active and taking care of your health!

Irritability

One of the DSM-5 symptoms to diagnose major depressive disorder is irritability, however, it's not always necessarily linked to depression. Irritability is defined as a low tolerance for anger or frustration, and studies have shown that perimenopausal women complain over 40%

more often about irritability than premenopausal women (Bromberger et al., 2003).

In society, being irritable is typically waved away, as "being a cranky pants" or "grouchy", but irritability really decreases the quality of life and should be taken as seriously as depression. Unfortunately, little effort is put into identifying the underlying reasons that predispose perimenopausal women to irritability. Irritability is typically considered just a symptom of depression, or a consequence of sleep deprivation.

One of the few studies that looked into irritability showed that women who had less variation in their estradiol levels, more frequent VMS or who were younger reported more irritability, independent of depression of any severity. It also associated greater estradiol variability with more depressive symptoms. These are important findings, as they suggest that the suppression of estradiol variability might improve depressed mood, but it doesn't help with irritability.

Estrogen supplementation has shown to help with depression, but it might worsen or at least not have an effect on alleviating irritability. Taken together, these studies suggest that depression and irritability might have different underlying mechanisms. So maybe for a long time we have been bundling irritability and depression together, when in fact, we should have been treating them separately.

Childhood Trauma and Menopause

Perhaps the most significant part of our lives is our childhood. A lot of our traits and personality come from nature, we see a part of ourselves reflected in our children, just like we reflect our parents. Some traits are written in our DNA, but just as influential is nurture. It is during early childhood that we start forming our character, defining who we are going to be for the rest of our life. It is no surprise then, that traumatic events during these formative years have such a long-lasting ripple effect, that can come back to haunt us later in life.

But how can something that happened forty or fifty years ago, affect our health so many years later? It has to do with inflammation, which is how our bodies respond to harmful stimuli, like pathogens, toxins, and irritants that damage cells. Inflammation is part of our immune response, and its function is to eliminate the cause of the irritation, clear out dead cells and start the process of cell repair.

An important part of our body's defense mechanisms are cells called leukocytes, also known as white blood cells or T-Cells, even though there are several more different types. These cells are like a microscopic army that activates when a pathogen attacks our body. It does this using a protein called interleukin 6, or IL-6 for short. Once a white blood cell detects something that isn't supposed to be there, it sounds an alarm by releasing IL-6, causing other immune cells to swarm and attack the intruder.

This alarm signal tells other tissues to join in the fight, which they do by dilating the blood vessels near the affected area. This increases blood flow and raises the temperature, which in turn causes leakage of blood plasma proteins into the tissue. These alarm proteins are released in situations of elevated stress, as part of the fight-or flight response.

So, imagine what would happen if this alarm was ringing all the time. Not as loudly as if there was an actual attack going on, but like a permanent background noise. Studies are linking early childhood trauma with increased levels of alarm proteins in perimenopausal and postmenopausal women. The exact mechanism that causes this correlation is not known, but their presence causes low level inflammation throughout the body that never quite goes away.

Most importantly, IL-6 is capable of crossing the blood-brain barrier, a layer of tissue that acts as the last line of defense protecting our brain. Once the IL-6 crosses into our brain, guess where it goes? Straight into the hypothalamus, there IL-6 does its thing, causes inflammation, changing the body's temperature set point, contributing to VMS and therefore to sleepless nights and depression.

Social Support, Stressful Events, and Menopause Symptoms

So far, we have discussed the multiple ways in which menopause tortures women with a wide array of symptoms, which are believed to be the result of hormonal fluctuations during the transition. VMS being the most frequent. However, while all women go through these hormonal changes, not all report suffering from VMS. 70% of women report experiencing hot flashes at some point during menopause (Gold et al., 2011), this means that there's a 30% chance of not experiencing VMS at all depending on a multitude of factors, such as diet, BMI or body mass index, and activity levels.

Even within that majority of women who experience VMS, the experience varies greatly in severity and frequency. Given how important VMS is in the Domino Effect Theory, it is important to understand the factors that go into the prevalence and severity of hot flashes, so that women are better equipped to deal with their transition.

We talked about how physiological stressors are directly linked to increased levels of cortisol and other hormones that suppress the immune system, cause inflammation and a cascade of events that worsen the frequency and severity of menopause symptoms. But psychological stress also has a similar effect, even if the cause and mechanism for this association is unclear.

Different social and economic factors seem to have an effect in VMS, such as ethnicity, housing, and socioeconomic condition. But perhaps the variable that connects all these factors is psychological stress, as women in different walks of life, cultures, or countries will have very a very different set of psychological stressors.

A factor that is often underestimated is the importance of having a strong support system, including a strong social network, throughout the menopausal transition. Having these tools available may help reduce the frequency and severity of symptoms, even if it is not completely clear exactly how these social ties work to improve health and well-being.

One explanation is that the perception of stress is just as important as the actual physical stressor, so having high levels of support might help lessen the perceived negative effects of stress. However, studies in this matter, have not found any direct links between increased social support and decreased symptoms. It is rather suggested that a woman's psychological reaction to the stressful event has the largest effect on VMS frequency, and it is a lack of support mechanisms that increased the perceived stress and therefore the symptoms. This means that women who see themselves as more resilient, when experiencing a stressful event, were less upset by it, and experienced fewer menopause symptoms.

The coincidence of life-changing events with menopause is inevitable. Since this coincidence is somewhat a product of our current social norms, which are unlikely to change soon, means that one way of tackling the emotional burden of midlife, could be changing our attitude towards aging.

Cultures that revere age instead of fearing it, like traditional East Asian societies, have less severe menopause symptoms. A similar effect happens in women that report seeing menopause as empowering. Such as women who now find themselves as finally rid of extremely painful lifelong menstrual periods. Women who have followed health protocols that allow their mental acumen to now peak, as they have care to divert energy from the ovaries to the many other life supporting organs[2].

That maybe reasonably rare breed of women who do not define themselves in terms of being physically childbearing. Women whose role models are older, even much older women. So perhaps it is a positive attitude, maybe honed by other incidents, or sharpened by knowledge and insight, that has the most powerful effect in dealing

---

[2] Read more about this in my upcoming book, The Miracle of Aging, forthcoming in November 2022.

with stress, and it is much easier to stay positive when you feel supported and surrounded by love.

Tips on How to Deal with Stress: Mindfulness

Stress is a fact of life, there is ample research on how chronic stress, both physiological and psychological, can have serious negative consequences for health. Despite the ample research available on the subject, there are few studies focusing on the experiences of midlife women.

Some of the few studies that do exist are showing interesting results. Women who experienced situations that caused them to feel helpless, overwhelmed, or fearful have a higher body mass index, more chronic illness, depressive symptoms, and greater sleep disturbances than those without these stressors.

It is vital then, to not only treat the physiological sources of stress, but also find constructive ways to lower the psychological stress. We already discussed how, having a strong support system is important, to diminish our perceived stress levels, but perhaps a more holistic approach is through what's called Mindfulness-Based Stress Reduction or MBSR.

Mindfulness can be defined as paying non-judgmental attention to the present moment. The crucial relevance of this precept is self-evident when we consider that most physical and spiritual hardships, including menopause symptoms, require that we judge ourselves as being in pain, distressed, or otherwise unwell. If we see ourselves as suffering, unworthy, neglected, outcast, misunderstood, unwanted, no treatment or medication will ever work, this is called the nocebo effect. It is the opposite of the placebo effect, and it's said to occur when our negative expectations regarding our condition or a treatment, cause the treatment to have a more negative effect than it otherwise would have.

Mindfulness is thought to involve several complex processes in the brain, including attentional control, emotion regulation, and self-awareness. Although the underlying science behind it is still at a very early stage, there are already some fascinating results that begin to showcase the effects of mindfulness on mental health, stress, and resilience. Individuals who self-reported as more mindful, meaning that they had a greater disposition to self-awareness, generally reported lower levels of perceived stress.

Mindfulness-Based Stress Reduction is a clinical program to facilitate adaptation to medical illness. It has been used to assist people with stress, anxiety, depression, and pain. MBSR is a combination of meditation, body awareness exercises, yoga, and therapy, that seeks to explore and change patterns of behavior, thought, feeling and action.

The best part of MBSR is that there is actual evidence of its effectiveness, as there has been widespread use of this approach within medical settings in the last 20 years. A typical MBSR program has a duration of eight weeks, with the goal of helping the patient pay full attention to the present moment in a non-judgmental, accepting way.

In a randomized study carried out in women experiencing menopausal symptoms, MBSR has shown promise for both reducing difficulty with hot flashes and improving quality of life. The results of the study showed short term improvement after three months, but also a persisting effect even one year after completing the program. Keep in mind that training oneself to be mindful is a life-long journey that requires consistency in its application!

Our understanding of the exact physiological mechanisms of mindfulness-based interventions is still very limited. However, recent studies have reported that MBSR training results in a smaller post-stress inflammatory response, including lower levels of IL-6. These findings also suggest that mindfulness interventions affect both the inflammatory and epigenetic mechanisms, that link severe VMS with age-related changes in genes that increase the risk of cancer and premature aging.

The results of this and other studies propose that mindfulness facilitates developing a more accepting, even-tempered state of being that helps decrease our body's overreaction to stressors. There is statistical evidence that MBSR causes an important reduction in cortisol levels. This allows a reduction in the degree to which vasomotor and physical symptoms are experienced as problematic or bothersome.

In other words, by dampening the perceived severity of symptoms, MBSR also reduces the perceived level of stress. And as we discussed previously, even perceived stress lowers the threshold of our thermal regulation mechanisms. A reduction in our perception of stress also reduces the frequency and severity of hot flashes, and since hot flashes are the first domino to fall, sleep, depression, and irritability are improved.

We live in a moment in time in which a basic google search can reveal alarming facts about illness or symptoms of menopause. Also, very few healthcare practitioners are psychologically and spiritually equipped to provide a truly holistic care, or even have the time or disposition to do so. It is easy to fall into a pitfall of despair, and negative focus can become a daily habit.

Maybe an eight-week mindfulness retreat is not an option for everybody, but it doesn't matter. The results of these studies teach us something very significant. That the best we can do to reduce stress and the severity of our symptoms, is to stop focusing on the negative aspects, the hardships, and the momentary discomfort. Instead, to rather acknowledge the changes we're going through and not let them rain on our parade.

So, surround yourself with a strong support mechanism, find comfort and understanding in friends and family. Focus on improving your mind-body connection, realize that both are just as essential and must work together to maintain your health and happiness. Work on keeping both as healthy as possible. Be mindful, eat healthy, exercise, and seek the right help when needed are foundational to any medical treatment that might have to be provided.

Even if hormone therapy or cognitive-behavioral therapy are not your thing, just the act of talking to someone, the feeling of taking action, can give the sense of control that we need to reduce our perceived stress levels. So, take control, and define your own reality!

Chapter 2:

GI Disorders (and Nutrition) Treat Your Gut Your Brain, and What are you Putting Into it?

The brain is the most important organ in the body. At least that is what your brain wants you to think. But when your gut tells you something is wrong, you know who you should listen to. The gut not only has huge influence over our brain. The gut's say in the body has a much greater reach, it is splendidly vigilant, and its influence is more ever present than what the brain gives it credit for.

Our gastrointestinal or GI tract is over 30 feet (10 meters) long from beginning to end and is home to over four thousand different strains of bacteria, with key roles in maintaining immune health and metabolism. It is divided in upper GI tract that includes our mouth, pharynx, esophagus stomach and duodenum; and the lower GI tract, comprised of our small and large intestines, it is also known as the gut.

A very important part of our digestive system that is often overlooked is the gut microbiota, or microbiome. It is a collection of bacteria, fungi, and other microbes that lives in our gut, they help us break down food into more digestible compounds. These bacteria outnumber the cells in our body by a factor of ten, yet only account for about 4 lbs. (1.8 kg), of our total body weight. It is considered a symbiotic organ that helps maintain a normal metabolic, immune, and hormonal health.

Gut bacteria manufacture vitamin K, which plays a key role in blood coagulation and controls the absorption of calcium into bones and other tissues. They also affect how our food is digested.

Gut bacteria help us digest certain antioxidants found in plants, called flavonoids, which, as we will see in a bit, have a very significant role in reducing oxidative stress, inflammation and in maintaining a healthy immune system.

It's hard to believe that a part of our body that has such a massive influence on our health is rarely talked about. Specially its role in the menopause transition, and how, if we just paid a little attention to it, it could help us so much to ease the severity of the symptoms.

The Influence of Menopause on Gut Microbiota

So far, we've discussed that the main trigger for most menopause symptoms is the imbalance of hormones, such as estrogen, and estradiol. That is caused by the depletion of the oocytes, and the resulting reaction of the endocrine system trying to compensate. But there are other physiological changes that can be derived from this imbalance that are not as obvious as slowly cooking from the inside every night. One such change is the composition of our gut microbiota.

The richness and evenness of our microbiome is used as an indicator of the overall health of our digestive system. Unfortunately, one of the major changes that come with aging is a lower diversity of bacteria, due to changes in physiology, diet, medication, and lifestyles. Often this results in an unhealthy gut environment that can predispose us to chronic, metabolic, and inflammatory disease. This is a condition called Dysbiosis, and it's thought to be closely related with breast cancer, metabolic syndrome, inflammatory bowel disease, and brain nerve diseases.

There doesn't seem to be a direct causal link between the reduction in diversity of the microbiome and the shortage of estrogen after menopause. Accumulating evidence indicates that the gut microbiota influences estrogen levels, not the other way around. Estrogen has an important regulatory effect on our immune cells, which have evolved to recognize and work along with our gut microbiome. Since our immune system keeps other kinds of bacteria in check, any hormonal dysfunction will indirectly affect the health of our gut, as harmful bacteria may compete or straight up attack our biomes. This includes the possibility of causing a mass die-off of bacteria, reducing its diversity, and by doing so, impacting our metabolism, and further impacting our immune system.

The estrogen that is circulating in our bloodstream is broken down by the liver, the resulting metabolites are excreted in urine and feces. However, some of these metabolites are picked up by gut bacteria, that reprocess it and put it back into circulation.

This is good news, since it suggests that improving the health of our microbiome can help women in the menopause transition reduce the risk of metabolic disease, and of conditions in which the chemistry of our metabolism is altered, such as diabetes; and immune disease, in which dysregulations of our immune system due to a number of factors, such as oxidative stress, cause it to attack our own body, or render it unable to respond to attack.

Studies show that variations in the expression of genes related to innate immunity and energy metabolism have been reported to correlate with gut microbiota composition and, by extension, metabolic syndrome. This is the medical term for the concurrence of obesity diabetes, and high blood pressure, that also may be associated with changes in the gut microbiome in menopause.

Species of gut microbes that used to work together in premenopausal women, instead showed a tendency to compete with each other in the menopause transition. Change in the substrate bacteria, like a reduction in trace elements, like calcium, caused by the decline in estrogen cause the proliferation of certain species of bacteria above others.

Researchers have speculated that differences in sex hormones may contribute to the diversity of the gut microbial composition, observing that progesterone could promote the growth of certain species. One recent study of sex, hormones, and the impact of the gut microbiome, looking to compare the biome of pre and postmenopausal women, found that the diversity and richness of the gut microbiota was significantly lower in postmenopausal women.

The difference in the microbiota included a higher abundance of *Bacteroidetes* and *Roseburia spp.* and a lower abundance of *Firmicutes* and *Parabacteroides* in premenopausal women. Lower abundance of *Roseburia spp* were correlated with metabolic and endocrine diseases.

Because of the onset of hormonal dysfunction, and its effect in the immune system that helps keep bacteria species in check, and working together in harmony, by suppressing harmful bacteria, the compromised immune system also is no longer up to this task.

The drop in estrogen has an effect in calcium absorption, which is a trace element that bacteria need to grow. This calcium deficiency can also result in increasing the risk of osteoporosis, one that is already significantly increased among postmenopausal women. Probiotics, have shown a positive effect on maintaining a healthy bone density at least, showing that it is possible to rehabilitate our good bacteria back to health.

Taken together, these findings show that gut microbiota certainly changes states before and after menopause, which might contribute to the many GI tract discomforts during menopause and the potential risk of diseases, which carry over to post menopause. However, the use of probiotics and maintaining a healthy, clean, and balanced GI environment at all times, can help prevent potential risks.

Gut Permeability, Inflammation, and Bone Density

Usually, we think that our stomach takes care of digestion and that our intestines, also known as bowels, and sometimes, as "the gut", simply manages waste disposal, but nothing can be farthest from the truth. It is the gut's job to absorb the products of digestion (carbohydrates, proteins, lipids, vitamins, water, and salt) into our bloodstream. It does this by controlling the flow of materials through the epithelial cells lining the gut wall, which only let particles of a certain size pass into the bloodstream, while keeping harmful substances inside to be ejected.

This property of the lower gut is called permeability. In recent years, a state of increased gut permeability, also known as "leaky gut," has been receiving more and more attention in scientific literature. It has been proposed that this condition correlates with a number of conditions seemingly unrelated with the GI tract, such as asthma, Alzheimer's disease, and diabetes among others.

Factors like psychological stress, intestinal inflammation, and hormonal imbalances can increase intestinal permeability, allowing particles like food antigens and bacteria into the bloodstream. This in turn causes systemic inflammation, resulting in several health issues, including autoimmune disease, like Celiac Disease and Inflammatory Bowel Disease or IBD. Menopause also contributes in no small amount to inflammation, which in turn leads to increased gut permeability.

Recent findings seem to support the idea that gut permeability increases from pre- to post menopause and further suggest a relation between gut permeability, inflammation, and loss of bone mineral density, which can cause osteoporosis in middle-aged women.

Fluctuating hormone levels during perimenopause result in a decreased expression of certain proteins in the epithelial tissues lining the gut. This, in turn, allows for bacteria from the intestinal lumen to cross the epithelial tissues, triggering immune cells to produce proinflammatory cytokines, like IL-6.

The various mechanisms by which gut inflammation can accelerate bone deterioration are still under ongoing debate. Studies in animals propose that the inflammatory cytokines produced by the dysbiosis, or the disruption to the microbiome, and imbalance in the intestinal microbiota is the key factor affecting the delicate cycle of bone remodeling. This process is responsible for constantly renovating bone structure, and that relies on an appropriate calcium supply.

This is a good point to take a break and explain how a lot of medical research is conducted in animal models (sorry, PETA). Understanding the biological mechanisms behind many of the processes that happen in our bodies, including the menopausal transition, is very complicated, as there are multiple interacting factors that are difficult to isolate in order to study them.

Systemic evaluation is difficult in humans because of the multiple life factors that need to be considered. Age, diet, environmental factors like, toxin exposures, drug abuse; genetic background, and overlapping medical conditions, make it necessary to conduct studies in animals. Since laboratory mice and rats are bred in captivity, it is possible to control all these factors, something that is impossible in humans.

However, as laboratory rodents do not naturally undergo menopause, it must be mimicked surgically, usually by the removal of ovaries. So unfortunately for our furry friends, whenever rodents are used in research involving menopause, they have to be surgically modified.

In one such study, researchers found that mice with sickle cell disease, a genetic blood disorder, had increased intestinal permeability, resulting in alterations to the gut microbiome. This was followed by bone mass reduction and impairment of osteoblast function.

Calcium is the main mineral in our bones, and typically we only receive it through calcium rich foods, like dairy. Among IBD patients, reduced bone mineral density is associated with insufficient calcium uptake and ultimately malabsorption due to vitamin deficiency, caused by the inflammation of the intestinal epithelial cell lining.

The calcium in food is mainly transported to the small intestine and absorbed through the intestinal wall with the aid of the gut microbiome. Vitamin D has an immense influence in promoting calcium absorption and bone calcification. Research suggests that a deficiency of this vitamin could lead to a decrease in the proportion of beneficial bacteria. Therefore, vitamin D can prevent the development of osteoporosis by controlling the gut microbiome directly.

Osteoporosis is a metabolic bone disease characterized by a decrease in bone mass and deterioration of the structure of bone tissue. This condition causes bones to become brittle and susceptible to breaks. It can occur in both sexes, at any age, due to genetic or environmental factors, but it's most common in postmenopausal women.

Our bones are maintained by a balance between two types of cells, osteoblasts are constantly producing fresh bone, while osteoclasts destroy old bone, in a process called resorption. The gut microbiota is closely related to the regulation of bone metabolism, and the absorption of bone-related minerals. Although the exact mechanism by which the gut microbiome affects this cycle has not been fully discovered, it is clear that gut health plays an unequivocal role in maintaining healthy bones.

The Microbiome and Our Muscles

Gut microbiota also has a very important role in maintaining healthy muscles. One consequence of aging, in both men and women, is the looming threat of loss of muscle mass. This is a phenomenon called sarcopenia, and it happens in both males and females because of factors that include neurological decline, hormonal changes, inflammation, reduction in physical activity, chronic illness, mitochondrial decline, and poor nutrition. But perhaps the gut microbiome has a more significant role than we give it credit for, in this aspect as well.

Sarcopenia, also known as age-related skeletal muscle disorder, is still a poorly understood condition, even though it's the leading cause of falls, fractures, and disability in senior adults. Some studies have shown that a combination of resistance training, protein, vitamin D, probiotics, and calcium supplementation are effective for tackling sarcopenia, but there is still an ongoing search for more efficient treatments.

A possible source for new treatments can be found in the relationship between the gut biome and muscle mass. One study stripped mice of their gut bacteria and found that they displayed reduced skeletal muscle mass and a decrease in gene expression for muscle growth. However, transplanting the gut microbiota of healthy mice into the bacteria-free mice restored their muscle mass (Lahiri et al., 2019).

There are several proposed mechanisms for this. Some species of bacteria, like Firmicutes and *Roseburia spp.* may lower the risk of sarcopenia and other menopausal symptoms by compensating for some loss of endogenous estrogen. The detailed, specific mechanism that links the human gut microbiome and skeletal muscle loss is still being researched.

Another interesting association has to do with a short-chain fatty acid called butyrate. Although the role and importance of this molecule in the gut is not yet understood completely, it has been found to be essential in maintaining homeostasis. The main butyrate producing bacteria are anaerobes, bacteria that thrive in low oxygen environments. The link between butyrate and muscle mass was first observed because patients that underwent antibiotic treatment that reduced their anaerobic bacteria had a more aerobic gut environment that negatively affected their skeletal muscle mass.

This is good news, because we can stimulate the increase of butyrate producing bacteria through nutrition, specifically by increasing the amount of fiber in our diet. Dietary fiber is composed of indigestible plant matter, so we need bacteria to break it down.

Science still has a lot to learn about the trillions of symbiotic bacteria living in the human gut. Their varieties and numbers are astonishing, their importance is undeniable, and yet, more than 80% of the microbe species that compose the microbiome are still unknown.

Stress, Our Gut, and Pain

It is surprising how little we talk about the health of our gut, given how many midlife women seek healthcare for GI symptoms. One of the most common, and quite frankly, one of the worst is irritable bowel syndrome, or IBS.

This very common disorder of the gut-brain interaction impacts the digestive system, causing symptoms like bloating, stomach cramps, diarrhea, and constipation. A flare up of IBS can last anywhere from days to months. It is a lifelong problem, one that is very frustrating and has a big impact in the everyday lives of those who suffer it, yet one that can be controlled and managed. The correct diet and treatment will help control the symptoms.

It is not known exactly what causes IBS, but multiple factors seem to contribute to developing the condition, such as stress, and poor sleep; (you know, the ones that are super common during menopause), but also poor diet, and lack of physical inactivity.

Anyone can suffer from IBS, at any age, but it is predominantly diagnosed in women before the age of 35. This predisposes women to enter the menopausal years with unfavorable GI condition. There seems to be a gender-related component, since adult women report more constipation, unlike men, who more often report diarrhea symptoms. Moreover, gastrointestinal symptom severity in women fluctuates with the menstrual cycle, leading to the hypothesis that there is a hormonal component to IBS.

The exact mechanisms that link sex hormones and gastrointestinal disturbances are yet to be determined. However, it is thought that there is a component relating to the immune activation that acts through what is called the brain—gut axis. This is a path of communication going both ways between the digestive system and the central nervous system, directly linking the emotional and cognitive centers of the brain with peripheral functions of the gut. Those among us who are keen on observing the body's many functions will have noticed a correlation between emotive factors such as sadness, anxiety, depression, and GI health.

We will also have noticed that overall, the hypothesis holds that individuals with a well-functioning gut won't have major issues making good decisions. It is almost like the gut is more the brain of the body than the actual brain. On the other hand, it is questionable how well a person can reason if their gut is dysfunctional. Absence of GI diseases gives a person the right appetite for good mental functioning.

Gut permeability increases from premenopausal to post menopause, being directly associated with systematic inflammatory markers. Taken together, these results point to inflammation during the menopausal transition, as the main contributing factor to gastrointestinal disturbances among midlife women.

When looking into the link between sex hormones and GI symptoms, a study focusing on younger woman found that women with IBS who used oral contraceptives exhibited less abdominal pain symptoms throughout the month compared to those not taking contraceptives.

These contraceptives contain small doses of progesterone, whose job under normal conditions is to tell the ovaries to stop producing estrogen after ovulation. This small amount of progesterone prevents ovulation by maintaining more consistent estrogen levels. Without a peak in estrogen, the ovary doesn't get the signal to release an egg, which eliminates the possibility of fertilization and pregnancy.

This result shows that suppression of ovarian hormones through medication can help reduce abdominal pain symptoms. Another related study addressed midlife women that were prescribed menopausal hormone treatment. The conclusion was that women using hormone replacement therapy were at a higher risk of IBS compared to non-users (Ana et al., 2003).

To explain this discrepancy with the effect of hormones and GI symptoms between these studies, we can point to similar studies carried out in women without IBS. These studies revealed that neither menopause transition stages, nor sex hormones were associated with the severity of symptoms like diarrhea and constipation when looked at over time. However, there was a positive correlation between participants with higher levels of stress and the severity of symptoms.

In a similar study looking at abdominal pain, while younger women with lower estrogen levels and higher anxiety showed an increase in severity of abdominal pain, there didn't seem to be a relationship with other sex hormones and menopause.

Instead, other factors are being proposed as key components for elevated perception of pain, like stress exposure, including adverse early childhood events. We already discussed how stress is a major contributor to a wide array of health issues, like anxiety, depression, irritability, sleep disturbances, etc. The autonomic nervous system is an important part of the brain-gut connection, so stress perception can disrupt this connection, altering gastrointestinal function, and triggering or exacerbating pain and other IBS symptoms.

Adults with IBS also have other symptoms associated, that at first glance can seem unrelated. For example, muscle, joint and back pain, as well as headaches. These co-existing pains are more common in women with IBS, and they seem to be related to higher gut permeability and inflammation due to stress, predisposing women to unwellness during menopause.

We already discussed the critical role of stress caused by sleep disturbances and VMS, so it's not a big surprise that it also contributes to IBS symptoms. Recent studies seem to back up this claim, showing that reports of poor sleep quality significantly correlated with higher levels GI symptoms the next day. This creates a feedback loop, higher stress levels worsen the GI symptoms, which in turn affect our normal function, leading to other symptoms that end up creating more stress.

In a recent U.S. national survey, patients with IBS reported lower resilience compared to the general population. This is consistent with our mantra that "we create our own reality". If we believe that we are less resilient, then our symptoms will be worse, because our brain believes it. So, all the steps mentioned in the previous chapter for dealing with stress will also help our gut. And adjustments we can make to our diets and routines will also help.

Phytoestrogens and Aging

Living in the western world, we're so used to modern technology and pharmaceutical advances, that it has become our first go-to. Feeling bad? Pop a pill! We forget that long before pharmacies existed, we were getting all our medicine from nature. In fact, 80% of the world population, according to the World Health Organization (WHO), rely on herbal medicine at least for some part of their primary healthcare (Martins, 2014). And probably only very few replace the Pop A Pill! with Take Many Deep Diaphragm Breaths. That, together with certain yoga movements, can have effects on GI symptoms as well as on emotions undesirable for our health, among other, that can be downright miraculous.

Certain foods have medicinal and nutritional properties and components that we often overlook. We call these functional foods. We consume them every day without knowing; vegetables, fruits, whole grains, and legumes. These help regulate body functions and protect against diseases, such as hypertension, diabetes, cancer, and coronary heart diseases, among others.

One such food component are phytoestrogens, which because of their anti-aging effects have become the focus of research looking into skin aging and oxidative stress. Some studies have also shown the relationship between phytoestrogens and a reduction of symptoms in post-menopausal women, especially vasomotor symptoms, osteoporosis, and cardiovascular events, through their effect in the gut biome.

Estrogens deficiency in menopause results in the acceleration of skin aging, as it causes a decrease in collagen levels, a protein found in tissues, that promotes elasticity. A decrease in collagen causes the skin to become thinner, and decreases elasticity, increases wrinkling, increases dryness, and reduces vascularity. Also, estrogen insufficiency decreases the defense against oxidative stress.

Phytoestrogens are compounds that our body creates from precursors found in plants like soy, flaxseed, and mulberry. Since these have similar chemical structures to estrogen, they can mimic its effects in maintaining skin health, preventing premature aging, and helping stabilize the fluctuating hormone levels in menopausal women, thus reducing the severity of symptoms. Think of them as mother nature's HRT.

There are seven groups of phytoestrogens, but the main ones are lignans, isoflavones, and coumestans. Lignans are present in the films that coat cereals. They are usually discarded during the refining process of flours, which is but one of the reasons to prefer whole grains and unprocessed foods. Lignans can be found in plants and grains rich in fiber, such as wheat, barley, oats, beans, lentils, garlic, asparagus, broccoli, carrots, and some fruits.

Isoflavones are produced almost exclusively by the members of the bean family. One of the main dietary sources being soy. However, small quantities can be found in other plants, specially nuts, fruits, olive oil and beverages, like coffee, tea, red wine and in several medicinal herbs. Soy is quickly becoming a popular food additive because it contains high quality protein, healthy fat, is high in fiber and lactose free.

Foods rich in coumestans include peas, beans, and alfalfa shoots. There is evidence these they help reduce the risk of coronary heart disease and breast cancer. Also, because of their similarity to estrogen they help in alleviating hot flashes and depressive symptoms, while favoring renal function and skin health.

A factor that has explained lower menopause symptoms in Asian cultures is that soy and flaxseed consumption is much more common when compared to women in the United States, who consume way more processed foods and fewer vegetables and fruits. In Asian countries fermented soy products are an everyday staple of their diet, they consume an estimated 15-50 mg of isoflavones per day, compared to less than 2 mg per day in Western countries.

The reduction in estrogen levels, typical in menopause, often result in an increase in the rate of bone mineral loss. Hormone therapy, calcium supplements and other drugs, are used to prevent and treat osteoporosis; however, they might have some serious side effects, such as increased risk of thrombosis and breast cancer.

Phytoestrogens have estrogen-like structures that bind to proteins in the bone, preventing the loss of minerals from bone resorption. One study in Japanese and Chinese postmenopausal women showed that an increase in phytoestrogen consumption was associated with a higher bone mineral density.

Phytoestrogens have shown potential in preventing oxidative stress, helping prevent inflammation, skin damage and premature aging. Studies in mice showed that they helped diminish the production of IL-6, reducing the white blood cell response that causes inflammation.

There is evidence of a direct relationship between phytoestrogen and gut microbiota, by promoting the growth of beneficial bacteria. Studies in Japanese population suggest that early exposure to a diet containing phytoestrogen may favor the population growth and diversity of microbiota, however, there are no studies specific to midlife women and the effects in their biome.

How to Maintain Our Gut Health

Managing GI disturbances can be challenging for midlife women. Multiple social, biological, and behavioral factors are in play that may influence gut health. It is very important during the transition stage to be on the lookout for red flags, such as unexplained weight loss, bleeding, iron deficiency (anemia), sudden shifts in bowel habits or inflammation. Also, special care should be paid by people with a family history of bowel or ovarian cancer. Women over 45 years old are encouraged to undergo yearly screenings for colorectal cancer.

Perhaps the most significant factor in maintaining our gut health is diet. Many patients report that certain foods trigger GI symptoms, so different diet changes have been suggested to alleviate them. Dairy, wheat, fried foods, and alcohol are all products that are well known to trigger abdominal pain, bloating, flatulence, and diarrhea.

Eating behavior, such as the timing and regularity of meals, play a significant role. Individuals with irregular eating habits are more likely to experience GI symptoms than those with a more regular eating schedule.

Dietary interventions for IBS focus on avoiding problematic foods and certain sugars known as fermentable oligosaccharides, disaccharides, monosaccharides, and polyols, which are harder to absorb by the small intestine. This is known as a low FODMAP diet.

Oligosaccharides are sugars that are a component in dietary fiber, they can't be absorbed by humans, as we lack the enzymes to digest them, so they're fermented by our gut bacteria, producing gas, which must come out as flatulence. Oligosaccharides can be found in a wide array of food, but they are most heavily concentrated in breads, cereals, pasta, and legumes.

Disaccharides are carbohydrates composed of two monosaccharides, or simple sugars, hence the di- prefix. For purposes of the FODMAP diet, it specifically refers to one particular disaccharide, namely lactose. We are able to break down lactose because we produce an enzyme called lactose, however, some people don't produce enough lactose, so lactose arrives intact in the large intestine, where it is fermented by bacteria, causing pain, bloating, gas, and diarrhea. Some people are born with this condition, called lactose intolerance, but it can also be acquired by underlying conditions that damage the lining of the small intestine, such as inflammation.

Monosaccharides are simple sugars, or sugars formed by a single chain of carbon. However, the FODMAP diet is only concerned with one, fructose. Fructose is the main sugar present in fruit, and when excess fructose lingers in the small intestine, it attracts water and leads to distension. When excess fructose travels to the large intestine, our gut bacteria ferment it, triggering gas production and bloating.

Polyols are small-chain carbohydrates that are found naturally in certain fruits and vegetables or as additives in processed foods. The FODMAP diet concerns itself with two specific polyols, sorbitol, and mannitol. Just like with fructose, polyols cause the small intestine to absorb water by osmosis. Polyols that are not absorbed in the small intestine enter the large intestine, where they are fermented by gut bacteria, producing gas, pain, and diarrhea.

The low FODMAP diet consists of three steps, restriction, reintroduction, and individualization. During the first step, foods with high quantities of these sugars are removed from the diet for 2–6 weeks. The second step gradually reintroduces them while monitoring symptoms. This is meant to bring on changes in the composition of the gut biome, including starving out bacteria involved in the production of intestinal gas. The final step involves developing a long-term nutrition plan to maintain a healthy population of good bacteria.

The low FODMAP diet is very restricting, so it can be challenging during the first, more restrictive phase, which is why it is recommended to follow this diet with the guidance of a dietitian.

The foods that are restricted in a low FODMAP diet include:

- Dairy-based milk, yogurt, and ice cream
- Wheat-based products such as cereal, bread, and crackers
- Beans and lentils
- Some vegetables, such as artichokes, asparagus, onions, and garlic
- Some fruits, such as apples, cherries, pears, and peaches

Instead, meals are based around foods like:

- Eggs and meat
- Certain cheeses such as brie, Camembert, cheddar, and feta
- Almond milk
- Grains like rice, quinoa, and oats
- Vegetables like eggplant, potatoes, tomatoes, cucumbers, and zucchini
- Fruits such as grapes, oranges, strawberries, blueberries, and pineapple

If you're suffering from IBS or IBS symptoms, you should consult with a doctor or nutritionist before attempting a low FODMAP diet, as it can be dangerous for people who are already underweight or have other dietary deficiencies. But there are some basic guidelines, we can all do to improve our gut health, and you don't have to wait until you have IBS or other GI symptoms to start.

Improving Our Mood and Quality of Life

Physical activity has been demonstrated to improve GI symptoms in anyone, and especially in midlife and older adults who are more prone to those symptoms. It helps with abdominal distention, bloating, diarrhea, and constipation through its effects on colonic motility, improving intestinal transit and by improving abdominal muscle tone.

Available information about the effect of physical activity on midlife women specifically, is still very limited, as the focus of most studies is on young adult women with IBS. However, these studies show that adults with IBS that were physically active during a 12-week intervention that included walking, cycling, or swimming, showed greater improvement in symptom severity relative to the control group.

Follow-up studies also found long-term benefits in the physically active group, such as improving IBS symptom severity and quality of life, while reducing fatigue and psychological distress. Sustained and systematically implemented physical activity has superior results, as compared to being physically active in fits and starts, or only if symptoms have not improved. Yoga has also been proposed as a potential therapy for IBS management. Therapies involving yoga showed greater improvements in symptom severity, stress reduction and quality of life than the usual care or lifestyle maintenance protocols in randomized control groups of adults with IBS.

Pharmacological treatments are available for GI symptoms, this generally include laxatives and muscle relaxants. Some are more targeted to treat IBS, like chlorine channel activators, which increase fluid in the bowel to ease stool passing. However, all these medications only treat the symptoms, but don't address the source of the problems.

Non-pharmacological options are a little more well-rounded, they include nutrition counseling, stress management, training in mindfulness, sleep hygiene and exercise. Cognitive behavioral therapy is also recommended to help patients by addressing dysfunctional thoughts and attitudes and providing patients with coping mechanisms.

It's very rarely that GI symptoms would appear on their own, they usually flare up in times of psychological distress, together with sleep disturbances, fatigue, and pain. This is why a more holistic approach is preferable, than simply treating symptoms. A good start would be evaluating what we're putting into our bodies.

Killing 3 Million Cells Every Second, Leaving Only Dead Matter in its Path

Our cells provide the communication with the world, they are our myriad invisible eyes that sense and see, and our cells are also exposed to all, including the vilest toxins. While on our side, we have no appreciation for our mitochondria's heavy work in their many confrontations with enemies seen and unseen. Including right now as you are reading this book. We take our mitochondria for granted.

The mitochondria are the powerhouses of the cell. The process of cellular respiration breaks down glucose to generate all the energy that the cell uses to carry out its functions and reproduce. The mitochondria even have their own DNA separate from the rest of the cell, that is passed down on the female side, meaning that you inherit your mitochondrial DNA from your mother, all the way back to the earliest eukaryotic cells.

Given this vital function, and that there is at least one mitochondrion in each cell in our body, there is no question of the importance of keeping them working at their best. Healthy mitochondria are crucial to the central nervous system, to prevent neurodegenerative disease, maintain normal cell function, and cardiovascular health.

The mitochondria's role goes far beyond just generating energy for the cell. It involves maintaining cellular homeostasis as well as regulating several essential processes, including immune and inflammatory responses; and proteostasis, the balance of proteins within the cell, necessary to preserve its structure and function; the stress response, and cell death, which is required for cell renewal.

Since mitochondria has its own private DNA, it can do things that the nucleus, the organelle where the cells "regular" DNA lives, simply can't do. One such thing is producing a special kind of protein, called mitochondrial derived peptides or MDP's for short. One of these MDP's is called humanin, and it's used to communicate with the nucleus and other intracellular organelles, as well as with neighboring cells and organs.

Humanin, and other MDP's are metabolically active, being responsible for allowing the cell to adapt to stressors like disease, aging, and exercise. Since mitochondrial dysfunction is a key factor in a number of pathologies, including obesity, insulin resistance, diabetes, and fatty liver disease, it is not surprising that a number of studies are now focusing on these proteins as means of tackling metabolic disease.

One of the hallmarks of aging is the progressive loss of cellular homeostasis, the delicate chemical balance that enables cells to work and reproduce. This balance can be disrupted by accumulated damage from external factors like pathogens, and oxidative stress, which in turn causes increasing susceptibility to multiple chronic diseases.

The communication between the nucleus and the mitochondria is vital for cellular fitness and overall health of the organism. Traditionally, scientists always thought of this relationship as being mediated by the proteins encoded in the nucleus, but mitochondrial encoded factors are now taking the spotlight.

Particularly under stress conditions, MDP's can transfer to the nucleus and regulate the adaptive gene expression, playing a key role in slowing down the rate of aging and delaying the maladies that come with old age. However, the levels of MDP's show a progressive decline as we age, due to accumulating oxidative damage to mitochondrial DNA. This damage reduces the cellular capacity to dynamically adapt to stressors and increases the disruption of metabolic homeostasis, which can cause any number of metabolic diseases.

Estrogens, Regulators of Mitochondrial Function

We took estrogen for granted for so long, not appreciating all the wonderful things it did for us, until we started missing it. It regulates our reproductive system, skin health, even our core body temperature. It even helps mitochondria protect our heart and maintain a healthy nervous system, including importantly the brain.

Our brains are made of several types of cells, neurons are just the type that gets all the attention, only because they do most of the thinking. Another very important kind of brain cells are astroglial cells, or astrocytes. They are crucial for the homeostasis of the central nervous system, as they serve multiple vital functions, like transporting major ions and protons, breaking down neurotransmitters, and by releasing neurotransmitter precursors, and scavengers of reactive oxygen species. They also undergo complex changes as we age, in response to different hormonal mediums.

Ovarian hormones, like estrogen, estradiol, and progesterone, have very potent antioxidant and neuroprotective properties in the brain, promoting cognitive health and preventing neurodegenerative diseases. They have a positive effect in astroglial cells, aiding in regulating their morphology and the release of neuroprotective factors. It's no surprise that menopause, with the associated loss of ovarian hormones, has been linked to several pathologies, like inflammation of brain and nerve tissue, loss of mitochondrial efficiency, cognitive impairment, and a heightened risk of chronic neurological and degenerative disorders.

This is because hormonal changes have a profound impact in astroglial cell physiology. Through binding to receptors in astrocytes, ovarian hormones regulate numerous cellular, molecular, and functional parameters, one of which is humanin production. Studies have found that hormones increase humanin content within cells, and that levels of humanin production were lower in the hippocampus of patients that had been ovariectomized.

Remember the hippocampus? The part of the brain in charge of memory and learning. Accumulating evidence indicates that hippocampus is highly affected by hormone loss by decreasing the number of synapses and density of astroglial cells, which has been directly associated with the advance of cognitive impairment.

Humanin and other MDP's are of great importance in the role of regulating the aging process by the endocrine system. Long term hormone deprivation can lead to alterations in the hippocampal mitochondria, severely limiting the availability of these important molecules. In animal studies, mitochondrial membranes from ovariectomized rats, displayed an altered lipid profile, which reduced their humanin levels and distribution within this tissue.

In vitro tests, that is tests outside the body of a patient, using cultured astrocytes, confirmed that this type of cell is able to produce and release humanin, and that it is ovarian hormones that regulate this process. Estradiol and progesterone work on astrocytes through signaling that starts at the nucleus, membrane, or cytoplasm. However, estrogen and progesterone receptors have also been found within the mitochondria, which serves as clear evidence that they might regulate mitochondrial DNA transcription directly.

Studies in mice have found that depriving them of these sex hormones caused accelerated aging by slowing down cellular respiration and ATP production. ATP is the molecule that is produced by the mitochondria, and it is used as fuel by the cell. To explain this, it has been proposed that these sex hormones promote an increase in the size and branching of astrocytes, without affecting their numbers. These changes are accompanied by the loss of the homeostasis regulating function, which is one of the mechanisms by which the neuroprotection provided by astrocytes is lost, causing disrupted neuronal connectivity.

These studies indicate that long-term hormone deprivation promotes structural changes in the astrocytes of the hippocampus, correlating with reduced levels of humanin in this area of the brain.

In vitro tests show that ovarian hormones regulate astroglial humanin expression and release. This molecule, which is synthesized in the mitochondria, prevents alterations of hippocampal neurons. Hormonal changes cause alterations in astrocytes, that could impair their role in brain function and may represent an underlying mechanism for mental dysfunction after menopause.

A Mitochondrial Connection: Fatty Acid Oxidation and its Role in Cardiovascular Risk During Menopause

Physiological and biochemical alterations can blur together to accelerate the aging process, and with this acceleration can come heightened risks in menopause. One of such changes is an elevated risk of cardiovascular disease. Less than healthy lifestyle choices, like smoking, drinking, and being sedentary as well as other factors like age, sex, and genetics, also play a big role in the onset of cardiovascular disease.

In western countries, cardiovascular disease accounts for 30% of all deaths, and is the leading cause of death in women, with more deaths than all other causes combined each year (Tolfrey, 2010). Various studies show a growing risk for cardiovascular disease in menopausal women due to negative changes in metabolism and hemodynamic parameters, like blood pressure. So, it is no surprise that the impact of menopause is being considered more and more when discussing hearth disease.

The lipid profile, meaning the measure of cholesterol and triglycerides in the blood of women in menopause can already be altered as a consequence of the changes to the gut biome we discussed in the last chapter. Due to its role in fatty acid oxidation, which is the mitochondrial process of breaking down fatty acids, alterations of the lipid profile will also influence mitochondrial metabolism in several organs.

Taking a quick detour to body weight, increased body weight is an unfortunate consequence associated with menopause. Our metabolism slows down with age, but the reduction in ovarian hormones can also lead to an accumulation of adipose tissue. Estrogen regulates the synthesis of various enzymes that normally help regulate these fat deposits, as well as the lipid concentration in blood plasma. Dysregulation of lipid metabolism caused by estrogen deficiency is shown to result in changes in fat mass and fatty acid metabolism. This leads to the increased body fat and visceral fat accumulation that results in abdominal obesity. Dietary recommendations include higher protein intake (1.0–1.2 g/kg/day),[3] low-energy diet, Vitamin D, omega-3 fatty acids, antioxidants from whole foods, phytochemicals, and probiotics (Ko and Kim, 2020).

Returning to cardiovascular risk, our hearths pump every day of our lives, without stopping (hopefully), that makes it one of the organs with the highest energy demands in the body. That is why it isn't particularly fuzzy about what it uses for energy, glucose, amino acids, lactate, ketones, our hearths will literally burn anything for fuel. However, the cardiac muscle's favorite fuel by far is fatty acids, in fact 50 to 70% of the ATP used by the adult heart, comes from oxidation of fatty acids in the mitochondria (Lopaschuk et al., 2010).

Aging results in a progressive degradation of mitochondrial capacity in the heart. On top of that, we have to add the alterations in the lipid profile that come from the hormonal chaos resulting from menopause. This results in a decrease of the capacity for fatty acid oxidation, an increase in the storage of lipids in adipocytes, or fat cells that store energy as fat, and the risk of developing insulin resistance, diabetes, and obesity.

Fortunately, there are things besides hormone therapy that we can do to improve mitochondrial capacity after menopause, and in turn decrease cardiovascular risk. I'm losing count of all the different reasons to recommend exercising, in this case, it's been demonstrated to increase mitochondrial capacity in the hearth, and to improve other cardiopulmonary parameters as well.

---

[3] For protein intake by the means of meat consumption, meat from sustainability farming is recommended, e.g. https://grasslandbeef.com

Carnitine is a dietary supplement, essential to long chain fatty acid oxidation. It supports metabolism by helping remove metabolic products (waste) from the cell, it also helps recover skeletal muscle.

Other interesting alternatives include resveratrol, a chemical found in grapes and its products, such as red wine. It has antioxidant properties and is considered an activator of mitochondrial biogenesis. In a study, freeze-dried grape powder was given to a group of postmenopausal women for four weeks. The powder was enriched with phytochemicals such as flavones, anthocyanins, quercetin, myricetin, kaempferol, and resveratrol. They showed improvements in lipid metabolism, as well as reductions in oxidative stress, and inflammatory markers.

Mitochondrial Dysfunction and Liver Disease

Chronic liver disease and cirrhosis represent the 12th leading cause of death worldwide, resulting in the death of around one million people in 2010, thirty thousand in the United States alone, a 33% increase from 1990 (Lozano et al., 2012). The rate of liver disease increases with age, becoming the fourth cause of death in ages 45 to 54.

The mitochondrial dysfunction that menopause brings with the loss of estrogen not only affects the heart. Physiologic aging increases the likelihood of cellular senescence, declining immune response, and causing an imbalance between antioxidant formation and oxidative stress. All factors that greatly contribute to liver diseases, such as nonalcoholic fatty liver disease and hepatocellular carcinoma (a.k.a. liver cancer).

There are a number of changes that happen within the liver as we age. There is a reduction of blood flow and volume, as well as a liver function decrease of around 1% per year between ages 40 to 50 (Iber et al., 1994). For women, the challenges of liver disease are compounded by the role of hormonal changes that negatively impact liver health.

There are three types of estrogen. Estrone, is the weakest, but it continues to be made after menopause when periods stop. Estradiol is the main female hormone throughout most women's lives, and Estriol that increases during pregnancy. During the menopausal transition, production of estradiol in the ovaries shifts in favor of estrogen, that is still produced in adipose tissue and in the liver.

Estrogen plays a number of very important roles in metabolism and regulation of the lipid profiles. Within the liver, it inhibits the proliferation of stellate cells, a major cell type involved in liver fibrosis and fibrogenesis, processes that occur during chronic liver injuries. These are a type of adipose cell that store fat, and they become a significant factor in developing fibrosis, an excessive accumulation of proteins, including collagen, that can damage the liver.

Liver damage is in some part caused by our own immune response. Studies show that females have ten times greater expression of the genes associated with detection of virus and bacteria. Also, the number of cells of innate immunity are higher in females, as is the immune response to antigens. These gender differences in immunity are related to the binding of sex hormones to specific receptors. This heightened immune response in turn causes an increase of cytokine production, like IL-6, that end up causing inflammation of the surrounding tissues. This immunological advantage decreases during menopause, however, the levels of inflammation producing cytokines do not.

It goes without saying that liver health should be a focus of any woman approaching the age of 40, while only few women have Caring for My Liver as a top daily agenda task.

Another consequence of aging is the decline of important enzymes that help eliminate the free radicals that cause oxidative stress. These enzymes form come under a distinctive group, whose only job is the detoxification of free radicals. Superoxide dismutase, glutathione peroxidase and catalase are the key enzymatic antioxidants of this defense system. We will look at oxidative stress more closely in chapter 5.

At higher concentrations, estradiol has antioxidant powers, but as concentration in blood declines, estrone starts replacing it as the main sex hormone. This hormone shows pro-oxidant effects, contributing to breaks in genetic material and increasing oxidative stress in the body.

Aging livers have an increase in lipofuscin, a substance that is left after cells have been damaged by oxidative stress, acting as proof of the increased oxidative stress in the liver. Estradiol therapy has shown to help restore some normal function to these antioxidant enzymes. This immunological advantage in women also helps them slow down the progression of fibrosis, product of liver diseases like hepatitis C. Postmenopausal women show higher rates of fibrosis progression, compared to premenopausal women.

Non-alcoholic fatty liver is currently the most common chronic liver disease, factors that are associated with it include obesity, diabetes and dyslipidemia, an imbalance of lipids, like cholesterol. This metabolic disease has a higher incidence among women in menopause, mainly due to multiple changes related to estrogen loss, including decreased energy depletion, increased visceral fat, weight gain, triglycerides, and cholesterol.

So, the data is not looking great, at least in what concerns liver disease and the paucity of addressing this condition in the mainstream Western medical approaches. This has not gone unnoticed and shows that a specialized approach to liver disease is needed among menopausal women with chronic liver disease. Also, it raises questions about the benefits of estrogen hormone therapy in the treatment of these conditions. Any woman should have detailed discussions with her physician about the condition of her liver.[4]

Mitochondria and Redox Dysfunction

We've discussed several times the effects of oxidative stress in different bodily functions, but we haven't talked about how exactly does that work. As if heart and liver disease are not scary enough, it turns out it

---

[4] For non-hormonal approaches, Traditional Chinese Medicine: A Woman's Guide To A Hormone-Free Menopause, by Nan Lu, OMD, with Ellen Schaplowsky, New York: TCMWF Publishing, 2010, is strongly recommended.

also plays a pivotal role in the onset and progress of neurodegenerative diseases like Alzheimer's.

In chemistry, redox refers to a type of complementary chemical reactions in which one molecule loses an electron, or oxidizes, and another one gains it, thus reducing its oxidation state. These are called reduction-oxidation reactions, or redox for short. These types of reactions happen all the time in nature.

They most frequently involve free oxygen atoms, which are highly reactive, though there are other molecules that act as oxidizers, all of which contain oxygen, such as ozone (O_3) and Hydrogen peroxide (H2O2). All these molecules are renowned for ripping electrons off other molecules. In our bodies, these reactions are caused by peroxides, the name for any molecule with a couple of oxygen atoms, called the peroxide group; or by other molecules capable of donating electrons, called free radicals.

A free radical is any atom, molecule, or ion, that has an extra electron, causing it to be highly reactive and unstable as it desperately wants to pawn that free electron off unto the first molecule that comes around. One notable example is the hydroxyl radical (HO-), which occurs naturally in the body as a byproduct of metabolism.

Another name for free radicals is Reactive Oxygen Species (ROS), they're associated with cell damage, and they are also produced by exposure to carcinogens and UV light. Because of their reactivity, they can rip atoms out of DNA, causing mutations and cell damage, excessive amounts of these radicals can lead to cell injury and senescence.

Our bodies naturally have ways of dealing with free radicals, detoxifying, and repairing the damage they cause. When there are more ROS than the body can handle, that's what we call oxidative stress. That is where antioxidants come in, they inhibit oxidation, bonding to free radicals and neutralizing them, which is why fruit and vegetables rich in antioxidants are part of a healthy diet.

Sex hormones, like estrogen, are natural antioxidants, so during menopause, when these hormones start to fluctuate, women may experience increased oxidative stress. Together with a decline of neurosteroids, a type of steroid that helps with normal brain function, they represent a risk factor for developing Alzheimer's and other neurodegenerative diseases.

Mitochondria are vital in high energy demanding organs, like the heart, but the brain uses up as much as 20 to 25% of the body's available energy, making it one of the most energy consuming organs in the body (Bryce, 2019). Estrogen enhances mitochondrial efficiency and protects from ATP depletion by regulating glucose transport, and glycolysis, the process by which the mitochondria transform glucose into usable energy, in the form of ATP.

Calorie Restriction and Other Treatments

There are three types of muscles in our bodies, cardiac, skeletal, and smooth, every single one of our muscles is composed of cells called myocytes. Cardiac muscle cells are also called cardiomyocytes, they are adapted to work non-stop, every minute of every day. Skeletal muscle cells make up the tissues that connect to our skeleton, making movement possible, also they're the most abundant. Smooth muscle cells are responsible for involuntary movement, like the contractions of our digestive system that guide food through our gut.

Skeletal and cardiac myocytes are very rich in mitochondria, they need to be, as they use a lot of energy every day to allow us to move and to carry out the basic functions of a human being. But over time, this high density of mitochondria also makes them vulnerable to oxidative stress, as more mitochondria produce more ROS, which contributes to heart disease and the loss of muscle mass and function, called sarcopenia.

Sarcopenia is one of the most universal characteristics of the aging process, it is highly predictive of falls, disability, and all-around mortality. Sarcopenia is also correlated to poor quality of life and in older adults usually increases the need for prolonged social and health care. Since muscle is one of the tissues with the highest energy requirements, loss of muscle mass is often accompanied by gains in the amount of total fat mass, causing what's called "sarcopenic obesity."

These conditions promote a vicious cycle in which declining muscle mass reduces the resting metabolic rate, the speed at which our body burns calories at rest. Since our capacity to utilize energy efficiently is diminished, this makes physical activity more difficult, leading to the accumulation of fat, which in turn releases cytokines, creating insulin resistance and accelerating the loss of yet more muscle mass. Sarcopenia is also heavily influenced by the accumulation of oxidative damage to muscle cells stemming from altered mitochondrial function.

While hormone therapy and increasing the intake of antioxidants are effective ways of reducing oxidative stress, calorie restriction (without malnutrition) is considered the most powerful anti-aging intervention. Numerous studies on animals show the contribution of caloric restriction to life extension, but also in slowing down the onset and progression of sarcopenia.

Caloric restriction is the simple act of reducing our caloric intake without causing malnutrition. It has been widely studied for its effect on extending lifespan and its ability to delay the onset of many of the pathologies related to old age. Mitochondrial capacity declines with aging, this is linked to decreased mitochondria abundance, protein expression and increased oxidative stress. Caloric restriction has been shown to preserve mitochondrial function, by attenuating oxidative damage, decreasing ROS emission, and increasing endogenous antioxidant activity.

The benefits from caloric restriction emphasize improving mitochondrial function and reducing oxidative stress. Recent experimental evidence also shows promise in improving muscle architecture by regulating autophagy in myocytes, a cellular upkeep process that is vital for maintaining healthy tissues.

Given the high reliance of myocytes on a continuous supply of ATP, the impact of mitochondrial dysfunction in skeletal muscle is very pronounced. The increase of reactive oxygen species in the mitochondria results in mutations of the mitochondrial DNA that accumulate over time, causing muscle fibers to be less energy efficient.

Caloric restriction in mice reduces production and accumulation of oxygen reactive species in skeletal muscle, improving the expression of genes involved in repairing oxidative damage. Caloric restriction may also cause alterations in the fatty acid composition of the membrane in mitochondria, making it more resistant to oxidative damage, and less prone to leaking free radicals.

Another recent study shows that simply by eating fewer calories, we can stimulate muscle cells to increase the number of mitochondria, reducing the workload per unit. This helps limit the generation of oxidants by increasing the biogenesis of mitochondria in skeletal muscles, which can be interpreted as a positive adaptation.

How much should someone restrict their caloric intake to get all these benefits? Well, it's better not go overboard with it, as excessive calorie restriction may be accompanied by a number of unwanted effects, such as weakness, osteoporosis, and depression. Plus, developing an eating disorder on top of having to deal with menopause symptoms can't be fun. However, recent data indicates that even a slight reduction in calorie intake (around 8%) combined with regular exercise, still retains much of the mentioned sarcopenia combating benefits (Kim et al., 2008).

Oxidative stress can also be reduced by consuming certain natural antioxidants contained in fruits, vegetables, and vegetable oils; honey, coffee, tea, and cocoa; fruit juices, wine, grains, and other foods. Some studies have determined that some functional foods can work as a preventive treatment to avoid or reduce oxidative stress in the brain. For example, fermented papaya extract showed to be significantly more effective than other multicomponent antioxidants.

There are studies that show very high antioxidant activity in coffee. Interestingly, by comparing antioxidant activity in green coffee beans versus roasted, they discovered that the process of roasting further improves its antioxidant properties, as it produces strong antioxidants, such as phenylalanine and pigments called melanoidins. Some publications have reported that the values for total antioxidant content of roasted coffee are at similar levels as for tea, cocoa, and red wine. So, take your pick! These are all excellent sources of antioxidants.[5]

Reducing oxidative stress by eating right and lowering caloric intake is vital in preventing and reducing sarcopenia. The most effective strategy to combat it, in addition to appropriate dietary guidelines, is exercise. Physical activity improves mitochondrial plasticity, and turn over, playing a critical role in preserving muscle mass.

The cellular functions responsible for regulating mitochondrial turnover are cell division and autophagy, this is our body's way of clearing damaged organelles within the cell. When mitochondria become compromised, and homeostasis is not restored through autophagy, the myocytes in muscle start dying, bringing on muscular atrophy.

Regular exercise helps restore mitochondrial turnover, leading to a recovery of damaged or lost muscle. Without exercise, the loss of muscle tissue creates even more free radicals, increasing oxidative stress, creating a feedback loop that only accelerates mitochondrial dysfunction.

Chronic inflammation is another important contributor to sarcopenia. Levels of inflammatory cytokines, including interleukin 6 (IL-6), are higher in aging individuals. They highly correlate with decreased muscle mass as mitochondria have a significant role in the immune responses to protect the cell during times of stress, causing a systemic immune response.

Physical training leads to an increase in local and systemic adaptations. Significant reduction of IL-6 receptors in the skeletal muscle was observed in obese, elderly and physically frail individuals after just twelve weeks of regular exercise. Another recent study in pro athletes showed lower levels of mitochondrial DNA in blood plasma when compared to non-athletes, suggesting that a sedentary lifestyle correlates with higher mitochondria-driven inflammation.

---

[5] Another highly recommended source is Ka'Chava. Visit http://rwrd.io/2f71qhc for discounts!

To summarize, mitochondrial DNA that leaks out of the cell due to oxidative stress can activate immune response pathways. The production of inflammatory molecules, in turn, impairs protein synthesis and promotes chronic inflammation that eventually leads to myocyte death and sarcopenia. A process that is slowed down significantly by regular exercise, high levels of antioxidants and intake of the appropriate foods.

Chapter 4: Immune Dysfunction

On Fire Without Knowing it.

As we have mentioned a couple of times, estrogen provides beneficial effects on several systems. Estrogen so prevalent in a women's body, that a decline in circulating estrogen after menopause is associated with risk of cardiovascular disease, osteoporosis, cancer, diabetes, stroke, sleep disturbances, Alzheimer's disease, and cognitive decline.

Studies involving healthy women transitioning into menopause have found a correlation with increased abdominal body fat, elevated levels of triglycerides, cholesterol, fasting glucose, insulin resistance, higher body mass index (BMI), and increased blood pressure. This association could be due to the regulatory effect of estrogen in lipid metabolism, although the exact mechanisms are not yet understood.

This laundry list of interactions is closely related to the inflammatory conditions caused by changes to the immune system. Low levels of estrogen have been shown to mitigate the immune response and predispose to disease and infection and an increase of cytokines IL-1 and IL-6. This results in having higher chronic levels of the pro-inflammatory cytokines, as well as decreased ability to respond to pathogens or external stressors (Gameiro & Romao, 2010).

For the past decades, treatment has focused on substituting lost estrogen and progesterone with exogenous hormones, focusing mostly in reducing symptoms and preventing chronic disease. However, clinical trials have shown that postmenopausal hormone therapy is not effective in preventing stroke in women with an already established vascular disease. Similar results have been observed for neurodegenerative conditions, with the results of recent trials of postmenopausal hormone treatment to improve cognitive outcomes being inconsistent.

Although these results are somewhat discouraging, they do provide a better understanding of how estrogen benefits the brain, heart, and vascular systems. They allow a comprehension of the key role of hormones as potent anti-inflammatories and their role in the immune responses.

Our immune system is divided into two branches. The innate immune system uses genetic memory to recognize pathogens, these are like cops patrolling the neighborhood with a picture of the bad guy. This is what gives us long term immunity after a disease, or vaccination. The other branch is the adaptive immune system, this is more like a SWAT team that gets called in when the body is under attack.

The inflammasome plays a major role in the innate immune response. It is a multi-protein complex responsible for the activating pro-inflammatory cytokines. It is like the neighborhood watch, constantly on the lookout for bad guys and signs of microbial tomfoolery or chicanery. Not only that, but it monitors damage associated molecular patterns or DAMPs, which are like the 911 calls from cells. Once the innate immune system gets the call, it sounds the alarm, leading to the activation of the adaptive immune response that immediately sends in its shock troopers, the T-Cells.

Repeated or continuous activation of innate and adaptive immune responses, due to external stressors, or pathogens, can create the chronic low-grade inflammation, which is typical of aging. The presence of inflammasome proteins in the cerebrospinal fluid of post-menopausal women shows that the decline in estrogens has been creating a pro-inflammatory state.

Estrogen works its magic through a network of estrogen receptors throughout the body, of which there are two subtypes, alpha (ER-α) and beta (ER-β). This last one, estrogen receptor beta, regulates key components of the innate immune response.

Recent studies are suggesting that the menopausal transition is responsible for an inflammatory response by the innate immune system. It starts in the female reproductive organs and propagates to the brain, making it more susceptible to ischemic damage. The inflammasome, therefore, is a good indicator of the effect menopause has on the immune system. Increased levels of inflammasome proteins in the central nervous system is a clear indication of alterations in the cellular immune profile. Chronic inflammation associated with estrogen decline can potentiate immune dysfunction.

Estrogens have a cardinal role on immune and inflammatory processes, this is evidenced by the increased inflammatory responses to infection, and the increased rate of autoimmune diseases observed in post-menopausal women as compared to men. Also, variation of chronic inflammatory disease activity happens with the natural hormonal oscillations of the menstrual cycle, pregnancy, and menopause.

The irregularities in the supply of sex hormones predispose menopausal women to immune disorders, like rheumatoid arthritis, an autoimmune disease that causes chronic inflammation when the body's own immune system attacks soft tissues. This disease causes painful swelling of the joints that can eventually cause deformations in the bone.

T-cell response is also affected by inflammatory signaling, causing a reduction in their numbers, which can also be correlated with increased oxidative stress. All these changes cause a deterioration of the adaptive immune system, especially during late menopause in comparison to perimenopause.

The innate immune system is the first responder against pathogens. Its role is to trigger an inflammatory reaction, scramble immune cells and promote the maturation of dendritic cells that function as sentinels of the immune system that initiate the adaptive immune response. Macrophages are another type of immune cells, specialized in detecting and destroying bacteria by a process called phagocytosis, in which the macrophage envelops and devours harmful organisms.

The ability of macrophages and dendritic cells to phagocytize pathogens decreases with age. Dendritic cells begin to lose their ability to present antigens and are less capable of stimulating T-cells. The adaptive immune system is also down regulated by decreased hormones levels as we age. This results in decreased production of healthy T-cells, instead increasing the production of senescent, inflationary, or depleted T-cells that are less active or downright dormant.

All these changes are a natural part of aging, which makes it all the more important to help our immune system stay healthy before we start seeing the consequences, by reducing oxidative stress, and increasing our intake of antioxidants, including vitamin D.

Perimenopause: A Systemic Inflammatory Phase That Leads to Neurodegenerative Disease

The perimenopause is the first stage of the menopausal transition. These final years of a woman's reproductive life are associated with profound reproductive and hormonal changes that increase a woman's risk of cerebral ischemia, a condition that occurs when there isn't enough blood flow to the brain, as well as neurodegenerative conditions like Alzheimer's disease.

Although the line between them is often blurry, there are two very clear stages to perimenopause. Early perimenopause is when menstrual cycles are still regular, relatively uninterrupted, and the late transition, which starts when amenorrhea, or the interruption of the menstruation lasts at least sixty days, up to the final menstrual period. Mounting evidence show that early perimenopause is pro-inflammatory, and that it disrupts neurological systems that are regulated by estrogen.

Throughout previous chapters, we have discussed the effects of inflammatory processes in the gut, muscles, bones, and brain, and its relationship with oxidative stress. All of these involve molecules called cytokines, of which we're already intimately familiar with the one called interleukin 6 or IL-6. These inflammatory proteins are intimately linked with our immune systems, so it is produced in almost every tissue and organ in our body. There is strong evidence that, during the menopausal transition, the decline in estrogen levels drives a systemic inflammatory state, characterized by pro-inflammatory cytokines derived from reproductive tissues.

Estrogen is deeply involved in regulating mitochondrial function in the nervous system. The estrogen receptor ER-β has been found to exist in the mitochondria. Estrogen provides its neuroprotective effects via the estrogen receptors ER-α and ER-β. Inhibition of either of them reduces the mitochondrial modulation of oxidation, failing to protect against inflammation in the brain.

Studies are showing the major role of mitochondria in regulating the inflammasome. One of the mechanisms of inflammasome activation includes the generation of reactive oxygen species, leading to damage and the resulting release of mitochondrial DNA to the bloodstream. Mitochondria are responsible for regulating the activity of the inflammasome complex, and ROS produced by the mitochondria can worsen its immunological signals.

Estrogen modulation of inflammation in the brain, particularly the hippocampus, plays an important role in modulating depression and anxiety symptoms. Studies show that this role is performed through the mitochondria, and that it is ER-β dependent. The fact that ER-β activation provides neurologic protection, stimulates mitochondrial functions, and inhibits inflammasome activation, suggests it has a central role in the crosstalk between inflammasome and mitochondria.

The most common form of dementia is late onset Alzheimer's disease, one in five women will suffer this terrible disease by the time they're seventy. It disproportionately affects women, as two thirds of Alzheimer's patients are female. One of the possible explanations for this difference is that women naturally live longer. However, increasing evidence proposes that longevity alone is not the only explanation.

Brain imaging studies have compared perimenopausal and postmenopausal women versus age matched men. One of the discoveries is that as women go through menopause, many early indications of Alzheimer's begin to emerge. Reduced brain mitochondrial metabolism in the frontal cortex, gray and white matter loss and an accumulation of amino acids called amyloid beta, are tell-tale signs of the misfolded proteins that form in the spaces between nerve cells, caused by Alzheimer.

Follow-up studies indicated that systemic inflammation and the estrogen decline associated with perimenopause contribute to the accumulation of amyloid beta, a membrane protein for neural growth and repair a corrupted form of which can destroy nerve cells. Administrating estrogen to ovariectomized mice reversed the elevated levels of amyloid.

Estrogen also mediates protection against ischemic damage to the brain, this is also managed through activation of estrogen receptors ER-α and ER-β. A more recently identified member of the estrogen receptor family, is called the G Protein-Coupled Estrogen Receptor 1, or GPER-1 for short.

GPER-1 has been shown to live in the cerebral cortex and the hippocampus, where it binds with estrogens to generate strong protection against cerebral ischemia. It does this by up regulating cytokine receptor antagonists in the hippocampus, a factor that limits ischemic cell death after global cerebral ischemia. More importantly, by doing this, GPER-1 preserves cognitive function following ischemic periods by enhancing the anti-inflammatory defense mechanism of mitochondria in neurons.

ER-β's involvement in regulating mitochondrial function in neurons play a direct role in preserving mitochondrial structure and function. The receptor modulates the mitochondrial gene expression that controls biogenesis, helping increase the quantity of mitochondria within the neurons, that as we discussed earlier, improves efficiency, and reduces oxidative stress.

Ovarian Aging and Timing of Menopause

One factor that can aggravate systemic inflammation is the premature onset of menopause. Premature menopause is defined by amenorrhea, the absence of menstruation; increased gonadotrophin levels, a hormone generated in the pituitary gland that stimulates the ovaries; estrogen deficiency, and the cessation of ovarian function before age 45. Women that go into early menopause have a higher risk of dying prematurely, suffering some kind of neurological disease, psychosexual dysfunction, and mood disorders in addition to the risk of osteoporosis, ischemic heart disease, and infertility.

Early menopause is more frequent than one might expect, with up to 10% of women in the Western world experiencing ovarian dysfunction before the age of 45 (Broekmans et al., 2009). Autoimmune conditions can set off a reaction that destroys normal tissues, and cause inflammation, together with genetic factors, they're associated with early menopause and primary ovarian insufficiency. However, population-based studies indicate that these factors do not explain the majority of cases.

Apart from surgical removal of ovaries, premature menopause can be facilitated by smoking, exposure to toxins in the environment, and malnutrition. Androgens are steroid hormones that regulate the development and maintenance of male characteristics in vertebrates by binding to androgen receptors, they're also precursors to estrogen. Nicotine is a potent addictive substance that inhibits the enzymes that convert androgens into estrogens. Because of this, chronic nicotine exposure reduces circulating estrogen levels and can trigger premature menopause.

Inflammatory factors could also potentially contribute to ovarian aging and menopause timing. In premenopausal women, IL-6 levels fluctuate during the menstrual cycle, increasing at ovulation and peaking during menstruation. This is normal, as this cytokine plays an important role in follicle recruitment and ovulation and is one of the factors involved in premenstrual symptoms, like cramps and bloating. However, these cytokines can cause systemic inflammation after menopause, which are closely related to oxidative stress.

There's another proinflammatory cytokine, similar to IL-6 that has been shown to be closely related to ovarian function, it's called the Tumor Necrosis Factor or TNF. This cytokine is produced by T-cells in our immune system, which is why it plays a major role in controlling infections, rheumatoid arthritis, and in bone remodeling. It regulates the bone marrow levels and activates the precursors of osteoblasts.

Studies have shown associations of TNF with early menopause. Interestingly, risk of early menopause was lower in women with moderate TNF receptor levels, compared with lower or higher levels. These studies also suggest that TNF regulates the balance of ovarian follicle development and regulation via apoptosis, the programmed death of cells that's necessary for tissues to renew themselves, as well as estrogen and progesterone production. Mice without TNF had higher fertility, larger follicle pools and a greater number of cycles per 21-day period (mice don't really menstruate, they just ovulate multiple times per month).

Correlations between ovarian dysfunction and lower TNF levels have been observed in a few clinical studies. When comparing the inflammatory factor levels in women with primary ovarian insufficiency, chronic anovulation (when the egg fails to release from the ovary), and women with normal ovarian functions, TNF levels were significantly lower in women with primary ovarian insufficiency.

Other studies suggest that high TNF levels may be associated with infertility. In rats, TNF administration suppressed ovulation while promoting apoptosis and autophagy, the mechanisms by which cells self-destruct, in ovarian cells that produce hormones. In humans, administration of TNF at low and moderate doses significantly increased the number of these cells in the ovaries of in-vitro fertilization patients. However, at higher doses, proliferation was not increased significantly.

Collectively, these studies suggest that the role of TNF in ovarian function is complex, and that healthy ovarian aging may be the product of a delicate balance of inflammation signaling, as performed by TNF and other cytokines and hormones, requiring precise levels, as either too low, or too high will cause infertility.

Immune Changes and Postmenopausal Osteoporosis

Bone is a dynamic tissue formed by osteoblasts, these are cells that are created by the bone marrow, that themselves create the matrix that gives structure to our bones. Osteoclasts are another type of bone cell; they degrade bone to initiate normal bone resorption. Together these two types of bone cells coordinate mineralization and resorption, in a continuous cycle that goes on throughout our lives, constantly renovating our bones.

During our embryonic development, a cartilage template of the skeleton is gradually replaced by bone produced by the combined actions of osteoblasts and osteoclasts. From infancy to puberty, bones grow in length by the effect of growth plate chondrocytes, the cells responsible for cartilage formation; and increase in thickness by the deposition of new bone matrix by osteoblasts. The rate of bone modelling decreases steeply after puberty, as bones reach their adult size, however, internal bone surfaces continue to be remodeled by the action of osteoclasts and osteoblast.

Throughout adulthood, bone remodeling is kept in balance by the deposition of new bone equal to the amount that is resorbed. After reaching peak bone mass in our thirties, we start seeing a reduction in the number of cell precursors of osteoblasts, and in the number of stem cells from which these precursors are derived. This causes a decline in the rate of bone formation, which leads to more bone being destroyed than it is created, causing a negative bone balance. Over time, this imbalance can lead to the loss of bone mass and deterioration of bone strength, which in some people leads to osteoporosis and an increased risk of bone fractures.

Osteoporosis is a systemic, chronic skeletal disease that affects one out of every three women experiencing menopause (Johnell & Kanis, 2006). Its main complications are bone fractures that impact mobility, function, and quality of life. Aside from being painful, it can be deadly.

During the bone remodeling cycle, osteoblast precursors are recruited from the bone marrow to bone surfaces by cytokines and growth factors. These precursors proliferate before maturing into the bone-synthesizing osteoblasts found at sites of active bone formation. Once osteoblasts have replaced the bone that has been resorbed by osteoclasts, they will undergo apoptosis, but some will become entrapped in the bone matrix and become osteocytes, a fully formed bone cell.

All this osteoblast action requires a lot of energy, and when you're a cell in need of energy, who do you call? The mitochondria, of course. Osteoblasts accumulate mitochondria as they mature. Unsurprisingly, bone formation is therefore deeply affected by the metabolism of mitochondria.

Mitochondria do more than just powering bone metabolism; they integrate the many pathways used for signaling by a wide variety of biologically active molecules. Mitochondria create a cocktail of proteins that play an important part in the apoptosis of osteoblasts. Not only that, but they also contribute in no small portion to the production of reactive oxygen species, and they are vital in maintaining calcium homeostasis.

Systemic dysregulation of energy storage and utilization, like the kind that often come with metabolic dysfunction, or in chronic diseases, like diabetes, results in an imbalance in the bone remodeling cycle, leading to the development of skeletal frailty.

Malnutrition also causes bone dysfunction. In addition to bone loss, low BMI is recognized as a classical risk factor for osteoporosis, resulting from a decrease in both fat and lean mass. Sarcopenia is also typically observed and recognized as a marker of bone frailty that sharply increases after menopause in women with reduced bone mineral density and even more so with full-blown osteoporosis.

Fatty acid oxidation mainly occurs in mitochondria and involves a repeated sequence of reactions that result in the conversion of fatty acids into the precursors of ATP. This plays an essential role in the activity of all cells in the body, as it produces the energy that cells need to function. Since carnitine transports fatty acids into the mitochondria, it is essential to healthy metabolic function. In one study, ovariectomized rats were given a carnitine supplement, which showed protective properties against bone loss. This suggests that fatty acid utilization is key to the maintenance of normal bone architecture.

Osteoporosis, immune impairment, and up regulation (the process by which a cell increases the quantity of a cellular component) of inflammatory responses are often associated with aging. Estrogen has a major role in regulating the production of cytokines, like IL-6 and tumor necrosis factor (TNF), both of these have been shown to inhibit the response of osteoclast precursor cells. Human and animal experiments have demonstrated the role of these proinflammatory cytokines as primary mediators of accelerated bone loss during menopause.

The very same interactions between the mitochondria, immune cells, inflammation, and oxidative stress that makes these factors so significant for cardiovascular and neurological health, are involved in maintaining healthy bones.

The study of the interactions between the immune system and our bones, is called osteoimmunology. It is a fairly recent concept that emerged from increasing evidence of links between the immune system and the health of bone tissue. Osteoimmunology is a field of great importance to understand the interactions of these two systems and their roles in menopause symptoms.

Osteoblasts are critical regulators of the biogenesis of immune cells, as both come from the same source, the bone marrow. Multiple mediators of immune cell function, including cytokines, chemokines, and growth factors, also regulate osteoblast and osteoclast activity.

Estrogen has a major role in regulating the production of cytokines, and IL-6 is a key component of bone reabsorption through the activation of osteoclasts. Irregular production of this cytokine is correlated with oxidative stress that damages the mitochondria, making them less efficient and causing a slow-down in the rate of bone generation by the osteoblasts.

Rheumatoid arthritis, inflammatory bowel disease and other chronic inflammatory diseases, are caused by an increased immune response, which is known to induce bone loss, by the action of T-cells after acute estrogen deficiency. A recent human study demonstrated that T-cells and monocytes, a type of white blood cells, isolated from post-menopausal women exhibit a higher production of TNF when osteoporosis is present.

By regulating the metabolism of immune cells, researchers are uncovering novel ways to suppress inflammation and treat autoimmune diseases. Studies in animals showcase the ability of T-Cells and other lymphocytes to regulate bone homeostasis. However, it is a very delicate balancing act, as an overactive immune system that's out of balance can easily cause uncontrolled inflammation and start eating away at the very cells that depend on them to maintain healthy bone structures.

Vitamin D, Fighting Inflammation and Promoting a Healthy Immune System

To return to our earlier analogy, if we let our bodies age like a poor driving habit, leaving broken car after broken car at the roadside while we believe ourselves ahead, purchasing the newest models, many factorswill cause unfavorable changes in our immune system. We often hear people recommending vitamin C, zinc, and other supplements to combat colds and even more serious health conditions. And while this is in general not terrible advice, it is not the silver bullet most people claim them to be.

Under normal circumstances, our bodies maintain a balance between oxidants and antioxidants, and unless we have a serious vitamin deficiency, taking larger quantities of most vitamins will only give us a marginal improvement in our immune response. However, there is one exception, the one vitamin that can make a serious difference in our health, especially for women who experience menopause. To get a healthy dose, you have to stand in the sun for a few minutes. I'm talking about vitamin D.

Vitamin D is a steroidal hormone. Because of its antioxidant properties it plays an important role in calcium homeostasis and bone density, but recent evidence shows that it also helps regulate innate and adaptive immune responses. Because of these properties vitamin D deficiency is linked to increased autoimmune activity and infection susceptibility.

The decline of our immune system can lead to increased susceptibility to infectious diseases, lower vaccination response, increased autoimmunity, chronic disease, and a greater risk of cancer. This weakening of the immune system due to uncontrolled aging is referred to as immunosenescence, and it increases the rates of morbidity and mortality in the elderly.

One of the main physiological functions of vitamin D is to help maintain bone homeostasis, by regulating calcium absorption. Studies show that vitamin D receptors are widely expressed in immune cells, suggesting significant interactions with the immune system. Vitamin D and vitamin D receptor signaling play a role against autoimmunity and have anti-inflammatory effects, stimulating dendritic and regulatory T-cell differentiation, and reducing inflammatory cytokine secretion. This suggests that vitamin D can modulate innate and adaptive immune responses.

Recently, vitamin D has also been shown to produce peptides that promote antibacterial response by stimulating the activity of macrophages. Moreover, epidemiological data proposes an important link between vitamin D deficiency and the severity of autoimmune diseases, such as rheumatoid arthritis, lupus, multiple sclerosis, type 1 diabetes, and inflammatory bowel disease.

Interactions between virus and vitamin D also seem to be more complex than previously thought. Studies among HIV-positive patients, show that vitamin D supplements seemed to reverse at least some of the damage to their compromised immune system.

All these factors make very clear the importance of maintaining a healthy supply of vitamin D. There's currently a debate within the medical and scientific community of how much vitamin D is enough. While the U.S. National Academy of Medicine considers 600–800 IU of daily vitamin D to be sufficient for the majority of the population, the U.S. Endocrine Society recommends 1,500–2,000 IU per day (Pramyothin & Holick, 2012). Although toxicity is rare, it's best to avoid long term doses of more than 4,000 IU, however a dose of that size should be perfectly safe for most people, and even necessary for some individuals.

Chugging vitamin D supplements daily might not be necessary, as the sun is one of the best sources there is. Our skin hosts a type of cholesterol that transforms into vitamin D when exposed to UV radiation, which circulates for twice as long as vitamin D from food or supplements.

Nevertheless, you shouldn't go overboard with the sunbathing. Too much exposure to UV rays will create free radicals and can give you skin cancer. Clothing and sunscreen can block vitamin D production, although it takes very little unprotected sun exposure for your body to start producing it, as little as 8 to 15 minutes will do the trick, however this will depend on several factors.

First, the closer you are to the equator, the more sunlight hits the surface of the earth. Because of the tilt in Earth's axis, at lower latitudes the sun beams hit the earth more perpendicularly, having to pass through less atmosphere. So, the farther away from the equator, the longer you need to spend in sunlight to get enough vitamin D.

The most important factor, however, is skin tone. Darker skin contains melanin, a compound that protects the skin from UV rays, but also inhibit vitamin D production. Lighter skin evolved as humans started migrating away from the tropics, so that they could get enough vitamin D in higher latitudes. Age can have an impact as well since vitamin D production in our skin becomes less efficient over time. This means older people with darker complexion will need to sit in the sun a little longer.

Fatty fish and seafood are also great sources of vitamin D, a 3.5 ounce (100-grams) of canned salmon can provide up to 386 IU of vitamin D, 50% of the daily recommended dose. Other kinds of seafood rich in vitamin D include tuna, mackerel, oysters, shrimp, sardines, and anchovies.

For those that are not into seafood, egg yolks are a great source of vitamin D. But if you're more of a vegetarian, your options are very limited, as the only non-animal source of vitamin D is mushrooms. However, it is commonly added to other products, including milk or plant-based milk alternatives, orange juice, cereals, and yogurt.

Chapter 5: Toxicity

Our bodies are Temples, Not Waste

Disposal

By now, my dear readers, I believe you are intimately familiar with several concepts that keep popping up again and again. One such concept is oxidative stress, we defined it as the imbalance between oxidants and antioxidants, and we learned that it is responsible for mitochondrial dysfunction, neurodegenerative and cardiovascular diseases, and premature aging. But let's delve a little deeper.

All chemical reactions, in our body or otherwise, are based on atoms exchanging electrons with each other. Our DNA is composed of carbon atoms held together by hydrogen bonds, in which a hydrogen atom with a positive charge, attracts another molecule with a spare electron, which has a negative charge. The same force that makes magnets stick to your fridge, allows complex life to exist.

Taking a small detour to explain oxidation, the most abundant element in the Earth's crust is oxygen. It is a highly reactive atom, and because of this, you can find it bonded to almost anything, forming oxides. This is because it has eight electrons total. Electrons orbit around eight protons in the nucleus of the atom, attracted by the positive charge in the nucleus. Because of this attraction, all eight electrons want to be as close to the protons as possible. Think of it like gravity, stuff wants to be as close to the center of the earth as possible, unless there's something to stop it, but if there is more stuff underneath, things just pile up higher and higher.

Magnets have poles, positive and negative. Different poles attract, and similar poles repel. In atoms, electrons orbit around the nucleus, just like planets orbit around the sun. The closer they are to the nucleus, the smaller their orbit is, and the less space there is for electrons. Since electrons have the same charge, they repel each other, just like the negative end of two magnets, so in the lowest possible orbit, there is only room for two electrons.

Helium has two electrons in its lowest possible orbit, and since there is no more room for electrons in that orbit, helium is not looking to take on more, nor will it part with the ones it already has. That is why noble gases, like helium, don't react with any other atoms, and don't form molecules.

But oxygen has other eight electrons, after the first two sit in the lower orbit, the rest have to go higher. Because of quantum physics reasons, the highest possible orbit is left with space for two more electrons. This drives oxygen crazy, so it will do anything it can to fill up all that extra space. These are called the valence electrons, every element wants to have its highest orbit full, so the number of vacant spaces determines which atoms can hook up with each other. Since oxygen is desperate to get two electrons from any source, we say it has a charge of -2.

Some atoms have the opposite problem, for them it's easier to get rid of a few electrons, than get all the ones they're missing. For example, magnesium has 12 electrons. If we arrange them in their orbits, it has two in the lowest orbit, just like helium, the next few layers are all full, with eight electrons, leaving the remaining two electrons at the top. This higher orbit also wants to be full, but since it only has two, magnesium is happy to get rid of them, so it has a charge of +2.

Oxygen is in the market for a couple of electrons, magnesium has 2 to spare, so they meet up, but since positive and negative attract, they get stuck together, sharing those two electrons, and forming magnesium oxide.

This is a very simplified way of explaining oxidation, but the same principle applies to other atoms and molecules as well. Because oxygen did it first, whenever any other element or molecule receives these electrons, we say that it has been oxidized. And the element giving the electrons has been reduced, which comes from Latin and means "to lead back".

Oxidative Stress, Causes, and Consequences

When we breathe, we take in oxygen from the air, and in our cells, it goes through a process in the mitochondria called respiration. In this process, glucose from our food is broken apart, creating carbon dioxide and energy. The mitochondria store this energy in a molecule that the cell can then use to power all its different functions, called ATP. In the process of creating ATP, the mitochondria produce a lot of free oxygen atoms, and other molecules with a negative charge, collectively called, free radicals, also known as reactive oxygen species or ROS.

These ROS are not all bad, they are actually useful for several physiological processes in the cell that rely on having the right amount of ROS inside cells. Our bodies have ways of dealing with the excess of these by-products of metabolism. Hormones like estrogen, and other compounds, like vitamins, bind to them, making sure they don't go around stealing electrons from places that they shouldn't like cell membranes, or DNA.

However, environmental stressors, like radiation and pollutants, increase production of ROS. When there are more free radicals than what our bodies can naturally handle, they start oxidizing proteins, lipids, and nucleic acids, that they really shouldn't. This is what we call oxidative stress.

A large body of evidence shows that oxidative stress is responsible, with different degrees of importance, for the onset and progression of diseases like cancer, diabetes, metabolic disorders, atherosclerosis, and cardiovascular diseases. If there was a reason for your hormonal levels to be lower than normal, for example, menopause, then the risk for all these diseases would increase.

Since ROS are mainly produced by the mitochondria, this is usually the first part of the cell to suffer from oxidative stress, diminishing its efficiency. This leads to mitochondrial dysfunction, as they need to work harder to provide the same amount of ATP, leading to even more ROS, and all the inflammation, immune, GI, neurological, and cardiovascular dysfunction, and disease we have previously discussed.

When maintained at healthy concentrations, free radicals have several beneficial roles. For example, they are needed to synthesize some cellular structures, they're used by the defense system to fight pathogens. Phagocytes synthesize and store free radicals, to be used as weapons against microbes. Free radicals play a key regulatory role in intracellular signaling, in many types of cells. Endothelial cells and smooth muscle cells in the gut, cardiac myocytes in our hearth, osteoblasts in our bones, and neurons and glial cells in our brains. See how everything comes together?

Another beneficial, free radical busting molecule is nitric oxide or NO. It is an important cell-to-cell messenger required for a proper blood flow modulation, it is also a vasodilator, involved in preventing thrombosis, and is crucial for normal cardiovascular activity. In fact, that is why nitroglycerin tablets are used to treat chest pain in people who have coronary artery disease, as it breaks down into NO.

If oxidative stress is not carefully and strictly controlled, it can be responsible for several chronic and degenerative diseases. Oxidative stress can also speed up the body's aging processes and even cause cancer.

The onset of cancer is a complex process, it requires cellular and molecular alterations mediated by numerous endogenous or exogenous triggers. Oxidative DNA damage is one of them. Cancer can also be driven by chromosomal abnormalities and the activation of mutated genes, altered by damage from oxidative stress. Hydrolyzed DNA bases are common byproducts of DNA oxidation, they affect normal cell growth by messing with the DNA of cells, causing the mutations that are one of the main drivers of chemical carcinogenesis, the process that drives tumor growth.

Cardiovascular diseases also have multiple risk factors associated with them, the most broadly recognized of which are hypercholesterolemia, hypertension, smoking, diabetes, unbalanced diet, stress, and sedentary life. However, research suggests oxidative stress should also be considered a primary cause for many cardiovascular diseases

Oxidative stress is the main trigger for atherosclerosis, a cardiovascular condition in which a sticky substance called plaque builds up inside your arteries. Atherosclerosis results from endothelial inflammation, caused by oxidation of cholesterol by ROS.

Several neurological diseases are also linked to oxidative stress, as oxidative damage plays a pivotal role in neuron loss, increasing risk of Parkinson's Disease, Alzheimer's, and other forms of dementia; amyotrophic lateral sclerosis (ALS), multiple sclerosis, depression, and memory loss.

A number of respiratory diseases, like as asthma and chronic obstructive pulmonary disease, are determined by systemic and local chronic inflammation, which are also linked to oxidative stress.

Oxidative Stress and Vascular Dysfunction Across Stages of Menopause

Throughout this book, we have attributed the ill effects of menopause to a deficiency of sex hormones, particularly estrogen, brought on by ovarian senescence. Estrogen, by being a powerful antioxidant, prevents lipid peroxidation, a process in which free radicals steal away electrons from the lipids in cell membranes, damaging them. Its deficiency after menopause leads to increased oxidative stress, which in turn can cause damage to major cell components, resulting in the cell damage or death that leads to all kinds of illnesses throughout the whole body.

Estrogens inhibit inflammation by reducing the production of cytokines. When estrogen starts trickling out, the oxidative stress and inflammation, result in the aging of blood vessels, decreasing diastolic ability, which raises blood pressure. This, together with insulin insensitivity, increases the risk of cardiovascular disease. Epidemiological studies show that there is less cardiovascular disease in premenopausal women than in men, but at the same time, men have a lower incidence of cardiovascular disease than postmenopausal women. This is evidence that estrogen has a protective effect on the cardiovascular system.

Oxidative stress is the main culprit of most age-related cardiovascular diseases. The mitochondria play a role in the production of nitric oxide in the vascular endothelial cells. The activation of proinflammatory signals, the expression of cytokines, and oxidative stress affect the mitochondria, hampering production of NO.

In premenopausal women, estrogen helps reduce ROS production in the myocardium, the muscles of the heart, essential to preserve the integrity of structure and function in the cardiovascular system. This means they have higher levels of nitric oxide, protecting the heart and maintaining healthy vasculature. Nitric oxide regulates vascular tension and diameter. However, once estrogen becomes scarce, the oxygen free radical O_2-, reacts with nitric oxide to create peroxynitrite, causing vasoconstriction, a reduction in the volume of blood vessels, resulting in hypertension.

High concentrations of estrogen promote vasodilation, which aside from protecting the cardiovascular system, improves the biomarker us to gauge the health of vascular function. A study concerning healthy postmenopausal women showed that taking replacement estrogen for one year, helped to significantly reduce blood pressure, and low-density lipoprotein (LDL), while increasing nitrite levels.

The association of menopausal symptoms, depression, and quality of life with atherosclerosis and other cardiovascular disease has not been well studied. Nevertheless, depression has been identified as a risk factor for cardiovascular disease, with several epidemiologic studies reporting an association between depression or depressive symptoms and cardiovascular events. In women experiencing menopause with no history of cardiovascular disease, baseline depression correlated with an increased risk of cardiovascular mortality over an average of four years.

Vasomotor symptoms have also been linked to increased cardiovascular risk and mortality. Hot flashes correlate with aortic calcification and reduced endothelial function. Interestingly, it was the frequency, not the severity, of vasomotor symptoms that was associated with these pathologies.

One possible mechanism for the connection between VMS and vascular aging is the effect of fluctuating estrogen levels in modulating the synthesis and uptake of serotonin. This neurotransmitter has neuromodulatory, thermoregulatory and cardiovascular functions, so it's not surprising that antidepressants that function as selective serotonin reuptake inhibitors (SSRIs) have demonstrated efficacy in treating hot flashes and decreasing cardiovascular risk.

Recommendations to Protect our Brain and Vascular System from Oxidative Stress

The very definition of oxidative stress involves having more oxidants than antioxidants. So that is a very good starting point to mount a strong defense against oxidation. Even though the body produces natural antioxidants, these start to become scarce during and after the menopausal transition, so it is up to our diet to pick up the slack. The antioxidants in our diets are the main contributors to our defenses against oxidation.

There are plenty of different supplements available that present themselves as being rich in antioxidants. Your local pharmacy or grocery store probably has an entire aisle full of colorful bottles of pills, gummies, drops, and powders. All kinds of different products, like resveratrol, green tea extracts, and even things with unpronounceable names, that you'll need to look up in articles in the references section of this book. There are also all kind of multivitamins, even some that are specifically marketed for menopausal women.

While there is nothing wrong per se with all of these, most of these nutrients are not going to be absorbed by our body and will just end up making some very expensive pee. That is because since a lot of antioxidants are only soluble in fat, taking them in a pill is not necessarily the most direct way of getting them to where they need to be.

The best way to make sure we have all the antioxidants we need, is to do it the way nature intended. Interaction between the different antioxidants in our diet appears to be more effective than the action of isolated nutrients.

Here is where another important concept comes into play, the dietary total antioxidant capacity, or dTAC, is the sum of all the antioxidants consumed. It is used to quantify the accumulated effect of antioxidants in the overall diet. Studies show that higher dTAC values lower the risk of developing chronic diseases, obesity, and oxidative stress.

In practice, dTAC is measured as a percentage of antioxidant capacity, from 0 to 100%. One cross-sectional study in Type 2 diabetic women found that those who scored in the upper 30% of the scale for dTAC, exhibited between 87% and a 94% lower chance of suffering sleep disturbances. This same group was associated with lower anxiety and had lower symptoms of depression compared to those who scored in the lowest 30%. More interestingly, these results were independent of age, BMI, energy consumption, physical activity, blood pressure, medications, socioeconomic classification, and total hours of night sleep (Daneshzad et al., 2020).

Our brains are very vulnerable to oxidative stress, they have a very high cellular metabolism, which means they need to have a lot of mitochondria. Our brain is also an organ that is very rich in lipids and fatty acids, both of which are prime substrates for oxidation. Also, neurons have lower levels of endogenous antioxidants if we compare them to other cells with similar metabolisms. This vulnerability is related to higher levels of inflammation, and lower neuronal plasticity and signaling, all risk factors for depression and anxiety.

Sleep deprivation can also be a cause of increased oxidative stress. When our brain is alert, it has a higher neuronal metabolism, and needs to use more oxygen, which raises the rate at which ROS are formed. On the other hand, as we sleep, we increase the antioxidant levels, promoting brain protection.

Melatonin is a hormone that our brains produce naturally in response to darkness. Besides having an anti-inflammatory effect, certain foods may be related to increased melatonin concentrations. Melatonin helps regulate our internal clocks, and makes falling asleep easier, while also being a potent antioxidant. Being exposed to light at night can block melatonin production, while partaking in melatonin rich foods, like cherries, grapes, bananas, pineapples, and dark green vegetables is related to an increase in melatonin levels.

There is a class of chemicals that naturally occur in plants, called polyphenols. Fruits, vegetables, and particularly nuts and seeds all have high polyphenol contents. Because of their antioxidant properties, studies strongly suggest that long term consumption of diets rich in plants offer protection against cancer, diabetes, cardiovascular diseases, osteoporosis, and neurodegenerative diseases. Fruits like grapes, apple, pear, cherries, and berries contains up to 200–300 mg per 100 grams of fresh weight.

Other than proper nutrition, regular exercise is one of the most useful strategies for preventing cardiovascular disease. Even if initiated in later years, exercise contributes to high physical functioning and overall health, and can reduce the risk of diabetes, some forms of cancer and other chronic diseases.

Exercise increases cardiorespiratory capacity, reduces blood pressure, total cholesterol and improves endothelial function. The type and intensity of exercise is also important. Highly strenuous exercise, above a certain load or when performed by someone who is unfit or unaccustomed, significantly increases oxygen consumption and muscle utilization, which in turn increases the generation of reactive oxygen species. So, it's essential to not overdo it, and carefully increase the intensity of exercise as we improve our fitness.

The key is to achieve long-term, regular, and controlled exercise. Consult with an expert attentive fitness instructor as opposed to just following the bros in the gym. Dietary antioxidant and vitamins, from a functional antioxidant diet, can help improve cardiovascular health by both reducing the cardiovascular disease risk and preventing or reducing exercise-induced oxidative stress. It's never too late to begin exercising and changing your eating habits; and there is plenty to be gained in quality and quantity of life.

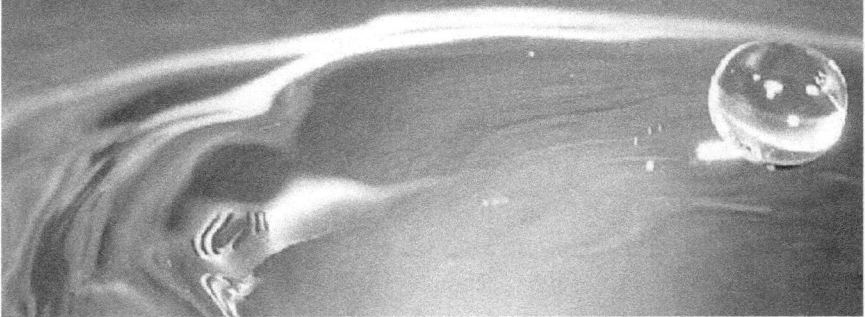

Conclusion:

Know thyself! Stop Ignoring Your

Better Half!

The many changes discussed in this book involve spiritual, psychological, and physical processes, which enable our existence by mediating emotions and the responses to our environment. We often take these three aspects of our being as separate, ignoring that the three come together and interact with each other to maintain balance.

Life gets complicated, it is supposed to be. That is what makes it beautiful and worth living. Even the most challenging situations give us the opportunity to grow, learn, and come out the other end, stronger and more resilient. Nothing stays the same, change is the only constant. If we stayed the same, we would miss so much of what this amazing, awe-inspiring existence have to offer, so why fear it? A butterfly wouldn't know what flying is if it had stayed a caterpillar.

Life is finite, and that is what gives each moment much more meaning. Each day we accumulate as well as let go, we convert some of our energy and vitality into experience and wisdom, and the side effects are the momentary discomforts of the transition. These discomforts are natural, and unavoidable, but they're meant to see you through to a new phase, not cripple you. That is rather the result of imbalances in our system, a disconnect between our minds and bodies that is making the transition worse than it needs to be.

Science is tool. Like a hammer in the hands of a child, it can be used to break things, so we learned to separate it from our more spiritual side, thinking it can only be used to teach us cold facts and numbers. But when in the right hands, a hammer can also build a house. In this case, science is confirming what we've always known intuitively, that our minds and bodies are intricately interconnected, and that our humanity is an emergent property of both.

We've learned so much about ourselves. We've learned that symptoms that we think are isolated are in fact just different sides of the same coin. Something as seemingly unrelated, as hot flashes and our emotions, are linked together by a complex web of hormones, nerves, cells, and mitochondria, so that one slight change in one, can upset the whole system.

The very tools our body uses to create life, ovarian hormones, have perhaps the most impactful role of all. Consider the number of processes that are affected by something so small. And yet our minds, that arise from the same interconnectedness, have an even bigger role.

Our minds rule over matter, and for a long time, we've let our bodies rule our minds. We didn't exercise because our bodies would ache. We ate greasy unhealthy food because our body felt pleasure from it. We smoked, and put things in our body that damage it, because our brains became addicted to them.

But in truth it is our thoughts that define our reality. If we convince ourselves that our pain is unbearable, it will be so. If our mind tells our body that we are strong and resilient, then that too will be so. Now our body is changing, and suffering, because it has been out of balance, in many cases for long, only now we finally have the label of "Menopause" as yet another excuse. Our mind has to step in and rekindle the connection with the rest of our being.

This is the final concept I'll introduce, neuroplasticity. Neuroplasticity is the ability of our brain to grow new connections, it could be in response to damage, as seen in stroke victims who slowly re-learn to control their bodies again. But most importantly, we create new pathways in our connectome, the map of all the physical connections in our brain, by learning new things, changing old behaviors, altering our perspective, and having new experiences.

Certain behaviors create neuronal pathways that strengthen each time we repeat them. So, the more we do something, the easier it gets, and the harder it is to stop. That is how we form habits, good or bad. So, the only way to get rid of bad thoughts and behaviors, is to create new, better connections in our brain, that are reinforced by good thoughts and good behaviors.

The physiological levels of estradiol play a critical role in regulating hippocampus-based mood and cognitive functions. Traditionally, the levels of this sex hormone have always been thought to play this role through the hypothalamic-pituitary-gonadal (HPG) axis, which forms a connection between the reproductive, endocrine, and central nervous system.

Disruption of the HPG axis has been linked to the decreased production of estradiol due to menopause. The abnormal levels of this hormone disrupt the hippocampal plasticity, leading to depression and dementia-related problems. However, it appears that some estradiol is synthesized by neuroblasts in the hippocampus, and from this finding, a new model is proposed.

This new model suggests the existence of a Hypothalamic-Pituitary-Hippocampal (HPH) axis. Based on the existing evidence on the signaling of estrogenic pathways in neuroblasts, the precursors that help form the central nervous system, it can be theorized that they might be responsible for the production of estradiol in the brain. This "neuroestradiol" is synthesized from cholesterol, as all the enzymes necessary for its production are present in the brain.

The regulation of neuroestradiol production resulting from neuroblastosis (which refers to the creation of neuroblasts) may lead to the establishment of a brain specific relationship between the hypothalamus, pituitary, and hippocampus through gonadotropin, a hormone that regulates ovarian function and is produced in the pituitary gland.

This new model would confirm that through neuroplasticity, the brain can adapt to eventually overcome even the lack of estradiol, eventually restoring hormonal balance. The brain is part of our physical body, however through willpower and discipline it can chart new pathways, even if the mechanisms behind this mind-body connection are still not clear to science, the power of our mind over the body is undeniable.

This means that many of the menopause symptoms can be overcome by training our brain into creating new connections, but to do this we need to start creating new behavioral patterns that stimulate neurogenesis, thus resetting the mind-body connection. What can be those new habits? Well, without further ado, here are 5 easy steps any woman can take to reset the mind-body connection:

1. Create a strong support system: Our body responds to stressors by creating inflammation and oxidative stress that cause a cascade of symptoms throughout the body. They end up interacting and aggravating the initial stress response. However, this response is also regulated by the perception of stress, so by surrounding us with people that make us feel supported, we are able to build up our resilience to stress.

    Don't be afraid to seek professional help. We all hate going to the doctor, and in recent years, there is a mistrust of the medical community. But if your symptoms are getting out of hand, if you followed all the steps in this book, and you're still dealing with depression, or cardiovascular disease, your life could be at risk. It doesn't have to be a medical doctor, or a hospital; therapists, nurses, anyone you can talk to will provide you with a sense of taking control.

    Do not be afraid or embarrassed to ask that your questions are answered, and to change medical professionals if you do not feel treated with the appropriate attention and respect!

    If there are any unduly stressful situations in your life, drug addiction, domestic violence, harassment of any kind, you don't have to deal with it alone. There are people willing to help, and that is something that can make a world of difference.

2. Be mindful: Pay attention to your body, listen to the subtle signals from your gut, your muscles, your mood. Nobody knows you like yourself, so don't ignore early warnings that there is something out of balance. Be aware of the changes in your body and accept them, revere changes in age as you revere the changes in seasons and greet them like a friend. Menopause is as much a part of life as childhood, so try to call to mind the prior changing patterns in

your life, significantly including those from very early in life,[6] and explore this new adventure.

Work on strengthening your mind body connection. Not everyone can attend a yoga retreat for several weeks, but it's not necessary. Give meditation a try, it increases your self-awareness, and reduces negative emotions, helping control anxiety. It also makes you focus on the present and gives you a new perspective on stressful situations.

There is scientific evidence that mindful meditation stimulates neuroplasticity, thickening the pre-frontal cortex, reducing age related memory loss, and improving sleep. Meditation promotes the release of important neurotransmitters, that help regulate hormonal levels, like serotonin, cortisol, growth hormone and endorphins, which also reduce oxidative stress and lipid profiles.

Remember that instead of being on a dead-end street heading at a permanent fatal condition, Menopause is the stage in your life at which to replenish, strengthen, and invigorate your GI, mitochondria, liver, anti-inflammatory, and antioxidant health, among other. In time strengthening these aspects of your body that are most likely to become endangered at this time is not much different than ensuring nutrition and care to an infant so that it can walk. So whence the anxiety and fear in which many become entrenched by their consideration of their symptoms? Evidence is aplenty that just as a toddler will eventually turn into a human that takes strides, women who successfully overhaul their systems in Menopause can experience not only cessation of symptoms, but importantly heightened creative and intellectual powers that they did not enjoy to the same extent prior to menopause.

3. Enjoy nature: More than half of the global population live in cities, Studies have shown that the risk for serious mental illness is generally higher in cities compared to rural areas.

---

[6] See my small book, Mindfulness Meditation, by Maria Ian, 2022, available at https://www.amazon.com/Maria-Ian/e/B09CQDZG1R/ref=aufs_dp_fta_dsk for this concept.

There are numerous reasons for this. Researchers were able to identify a definitive relationship between trees and stress. In the study at a lower level of tree density of 2%, 41% of participants in urban environments reported a calming effect. As tree cover density reached 36%, more than 90% of participants reported a stress recovery experience (Jiang et al., 2014).

Also, the benefits of vitamin D cannot be understated, it is vital for healthy immune response, reduces oxidative stress, and helps protect our brain and heart. And to get it, you only need to spend ten to twenty minutes under the sun. You don't have to move to the country to get these benefits, one short walk in the park every morning should do.

4. Be careful with what you put in your body: You are what you eat, there's no way around it. We've discussed the huge number of benefits of several dietary approaches including an antioxidant rich diet, so including fresh fruits and vegetables in your meals will have a major impact in protecting your health and reduce menopause symptoms. Coffee, tea, or wine are also excellent sources, although, try not indulging in alcohol, as it is a vasoconstrictor and stimulates the production of free radicals.

5. Exercise: If you have to pick only one piece of advice in this book to follow, let it be this one. A sedentary life will kill you. Every single symptom, disorder, or disease mentioned in this book can be prevented, attenuated, or downright cured, by regular exercise.

    You don't have to start running marathons or lifting weights. Even though there are added benefits to strength training, such as increase bone and muscle mass, any kind of activity that raises your heart rate will do the trick. Exercise stimulates production of endorphins, that have neuroprotective and antidepressant properties.

    Exercise stimulates the biogenesis of mitochondria, improving your metabolism, and reducing oxidative stress. It increases your respiratory capacity, lowers your resting heart rate, burns fat, and helps you sleep better.

Plus, you can combine it with tip#3, just 30 minutes three times a week of vigorous exercise is enough to radically improve your health.

The above tips not only apply to menopausal women, but everyone can also benefit from strengthening their mind-body connection, no matter the age, sex, or ethnicity.

Don't wait until your health is already in the decline before taking action. Even if you've always been a healthy person, the best way to stay that way is by being proactive.

I really hope that you find this book informative, and that it helps you make this transition at least a little easier. Remember, you are not alone in this journey, so try if you can help others along the way, medicine is expensive, but information is priceless.

Glossary

Adipocytes: cells specialized in storing energy as fat (Encyclopedia Britannica, n.d.)

Adrenaline: A hormone produced in the adrenal glands that plays an important part in the flight or fight response (Marks et al., 2013)

Amenorrhea: the absence of menstruation, often defined as missing one or more menstrual periods (Mayo Clinic, 2021).

Amyloid plaques: aggregates of misfolded proteins that form in the spaces between nerve cells. Thought to play a central role in Alzheimer's disease, they first develop in the areas of the brain concerned with memory and other cognitive functions (Robertson, 2018).

Anovulation: when the ovaries do not release an oocyte during a menstrual cycle. Therefore, ovulation does not take place (Hamilton-Fairley & Taylor, 2003).

Apoptosis: A type of cell death in which a series of molecular steps in a cell lead to its death. This is one method the body uses to get rid of unneeded or abnormal cells (National Cancer Institute, n.d.).

Astroglial cells: Also known as astrocytes, they are neural cells that provide for homeostasis and defense of the central nervous system (CNS) (Verkhatsky & Nedergaard, 2017)

Atherosclerosis: a condition that develops when a sticky substance called plaque builds up inside your arteries (National Heart, Lung, and Blood Institute, 2022)

Autophagy: a process involved in the orderly degradation and recycling of cellular components (Mizushima & Komatsu, 2011).

Butyrate: Also known as Butyric acid. It is a short-chain fatty acid produced by some types of gut bacteria when they break down or digest fiber (Mitchell, 2020).

Carnitine: a chemical produced by the body, involved in fatty acid metabolism (Bremer, 1983)

Cerebral ischemia: a condition in which there isn't sufficient blood flow to the brain, leading to limited oxygen supply or cerebral hypoxia and leads to the death of brain tissue, cerebral infarction, or ischemic stroke (Columbia Neurosurgery, n.d.)

Chlorine channel activators: medication used to treat constipation and irritable bowel syndrome. They work by increasing fluid, allowing for easier stool passing (Jentsch et al., 2002).

Circadian rhythm: the natural process that regulates the sleep–wake cycle and repeats every 24 hours. (National Institute of Neurological Disorders and Stroke, 2022)

Coronary Arterial Disease (CAD): The most common of heart diseases in the United States. Caused by plaque buildup in the walls of the arteries that supply blood to the heart, that causes the inside of the arteries to narrow over time, which can partially or totally block the blood flow to the heart (National Center for Chronic Disease Prevention and Health Promotion, 2021).

Cortisol: One of the hormones produced in the adrenal glands that regulates a wide range of vital processes throughout the body, including metabolism and the immune response. It also has a very important role in helping the body respond to stress. (Society for Endocrinology, 2019)

Cognitive-behavioral therapy: psychological treatment with demonstrated effectiveness in improving a range of problems including depression and anxiety disorders, alcohol and drug abuse, relationship problems, eating disorders, and mental illness. (APA Div. 12 (Society of Clinical Psychology), 2017)

Connectome: the complete map of the neural connections in a brain (Sporns, 2014).

Cytokines: proteins that regulate the growth and activity of other immune system and blood cells, i.e., IL-6 (American Cancer Society, 2019).

Damage associated molecular patterns (DAMPs): endogenous danger molecules that are released from damaged or dying cells and activate the innate immune system (Roh & Sohn, 2018)

Dendritic cells: immune cells that effectively link the innate and adaptive arms of the immune system (McQueen, 2010)

Dietary total antioxidant capacity (dTAC): the sum total of all or most of the antioxidants being consumed, which estimates the cumulative effect of the antioxidants in the overall diet (Pereira et al., 2021)

Dysbiosis: imbalances and abnormalities of the microbiota that result in negative effects on the host (Hou et al., 2021)

Dyslipidemia: an imbalance of lipids such as cholesterol, low-density lipoprotein cholesterol, (LDL-C), triglycerides, and high-density lipoprotein (HDL). This condition can result from diet, tobacco exposure, or genetic and can lead to cardiovascular disease with severe complications (Pappan & Rehman, 2022).

Dysmenorrhea: a chemical imbalance that causes abnormal contractions of the uterus, resulting in severe and frequent cramps and pain during menstruation (Johns Hopkins Medicine, n.d.).

Estrone: a weak form of estrogen synthesized from cholesterol in adipose tissue (Kuhl, 2005).

Free Radicals: reactive and unstable molecules, produced naturally as a byproduct of metabolism, or by exposure to toxins and other environmental factors such as tobacco smoke and ultraviolet light (Eldridge, 2022).

FODMAP diet: A diet designed to help people with irritable bowel syndrome, that is low in certain sugars (Fermentable Oligosaccharides,

Disaccharides, Monosaccharides, and Polyols) that irritate the small intestine (Veloso, n.d.).

Gastrointestinal (GI) Tract: The digestive tract is made up of the organs that food and liquids travel through when they are swallowed, digested, absorbed, and leave the body as feces. These organs include the mouth, pharynx (throat), esophagus, stomach, small intestine, large intestine, rectum, and anus (National Cancer Institute, n.d.).

Gonadotropins: peptide hormones that regulate ovarian and testicular function and are essential for normal growth, sexual development, and reproduction (National Institute of Diabetes and Digestive and Kidney Diseases., 2018)

Gut Permeability: the property that controls the flow of material passing from inside the gastrointestinal tract through the cells lining the gut wall, into the bloodstream (Hanauer et al., 2002).

Homeostasis: a relatively stable state of equilibrium or a tendency toward such a state between the different but interdependent elements or groups of elements of an organism, population, or group (Merriam-Webster, (n.d.)).}

Hormone: a protein that works as a signaling molecule for biological processes, that regulate physiology and behavior (Vigna et al., 2014).

Hippocampus: the part of the brain that plays an important role in memory and consolidation of information

Hypothalamus: the part of the brain linking the nervous and endocrine systems, responsible for regulating metabolic processes and the autonomic nervous system (Singh, 2011).

Immunosenescence: a process of immune dysfunction that occurs with age and includes remodeling of lymphoid organs, leading to changes in the immune function of the elderly. (Lian et al., 2020).

Inflammasome: innate immune system receptors and sensors that regulate inflammation in response to infectious microbes and molecules derived from host proteins (Guo et al., 2015).

Irritable bowel syndrome (IBS): a common chronic disorder that affects the large intestine. Symptoms include cramping, abdominal pain, bloating, gas, and diarrhea or constipation (The Mayo Clinic, 2021).

Leukocytes: A type of blood cell of the immune system that helps the body fight infection and other diseases, also known as white blood cells (National Cancer Institute, n.d.).

Lipofuscin: a yellowish-brown lipid-containing pigment that accumulates in the cytoplasm of cells during aging, that can be neither degraded nor ejected from the cell but can only be diluted through cell division and growth (Gray & Woulfe, 2005).

Macrophage: specialized cells involved in the detection, phagocytosis, and destruction of bacteria and other harmful organisms. In addition, they can also present antigens to T cells and initiate inflammation by releasing cytokines that activate other cells (Saldana, n.d.).

Melatonin: a hormone produced by the brain produces in response to darkness. It helps with the timing of your circadian rhythms (24-hour internal clock) and with sleep (Costello et al., 2014).

Menopause: the moment in a woman's life in which menstruation stops and is no longer fertile. (Shriver, 2013).

Metabolic syndrome: the medical term for a combination of diabetes, high blood pressure (hypertension) and obesity (National Health Service, 2019).

Microbiome / microbiota: a collection of microbes, such as bacteria, fungi, viruses, and their genes, that naturally inhabit our bodies (National Institute of Environmental Health Sciences, 2022).

Mindfulness-based stress reduction: an evidence-based program offering intensive training that seeks to help people with stress, anxiety, depression, and pain (American Psychological Association, 2019).

Mitochondria: an organelle found in most eukaryotic cells that use aerobic respiration to generate the cell's energy supply in the form of adenosine triphosphate (ATP) (Campbell, 2006).

Mitochondrial derive peptides (MDP): small peptides hidden in the mitochondrial DNA, maintaining mitochondrial function, and protecting cells under different stresses (Dabravolski et al., 2021).

Myocyte: the cells that make up muscle tissue (Baxter, n.d.).

Neuroendocrinology: The branch of physiology that studies how the nervous system controls hormonal secretion and how hormones control the brain (Fink et al., 2012).

Neuroplasticity: the brain's ability to modify, change, and adapt both structure and function throughout life and in response to experience (Voss et al., 2017).

Nocebo effect: A situation in which a patient develops side effects or symptoms that can occur with a drug or other therapy just because the patient believes they may occur (National Cancer Institute, n.d.).

Oncobiome: Gut microbiota plays a role in cancer (Hou et al., 2021).

Oocyte: an immature egg that develops to maturity from within a structure called follicles, which are found in the outside layer of the ovaries. (White et al., 2012)

Osteoblasts: specialized mesenchymal cells that synthesize bone matrix and coordinate the mineralization of the skeleton (Dirckx et al., 2019)

Osteoclasts: cells that degrade bone to initiate normal bone remodeling and mediate bone loss in pathologic conditions by increasing their resorptive activity (Boyce et al., 2010).

Osteocytes: osteoblasts that become surrounded by unmineralized matrix during bone formation; they make up 90–95% of the adult bone cell population (Schaffler et al., 2015)

Osteoimmunology: a medical field that studies the interface between the skeletal system and the immune system (Walsh et al., 2006)

Osteoporosis: a systemic skeletal disorder characterized by loss of bone mass (Golob & Laya, 2015).

Oxidation-reduction reaction (Redox): a type of complementary chemical reactions in which the oxidation states of a substrate changes by losing or gaining an electron, thus increasing, or reducing its oxidation state (Haustein, 2019).

Oxidative stress: an imbalance between production of oxygen reactive species (ROS) in cells and tissues, and the ability of a biological system to remove these reactive products (Pizzino et al., 2017).

Phagocytosis: a cellular process for eliminating microscopic particles, including microorganisms, foreign substances, and apoptotic cells (Uribe-Querol & Rosales, 2020).

Phytoestrogens: a diverse group of naturally occurring non-steroidal plant compounds that, because of its structural similarity with estradiol, have the ability to cause effects similar to those of estrogen (Yildiz, 2006).

Physiological stress: a state of fight or flight response, caused by intrinsic or extrinsic stimuli either real or perceived, which are defined as stressors (Agorastos & Chrousos, 2021).

Proteostasis: an extensive network of components that acts to maintain proteins in the correct concentration, conformation, and subcellular location, to cooperatively achieve the stability and functional features of the proteome (Clausen et al., 2019).

Reactive Oxygen Species: highly reactive chemicals formed from O2 (Hayyan et al., 2016)

Resveratrol: A type of natural phenol produced by several plants, including grapevines in response to injury, with antioxidant properties (Frémont, 2000).

Rheumatoid arthritis: an autoimmune disease that causes joint inflammation and pain. It happens when the immune system doesn't work properly and attacks the lining of the joints, called the synovium (Arthritis Foundation, 2021).

Sarcopenia: An age related, involuntary loss of skeletal muscle mass and strength (Walston, 2012).

Sarcopenic obesity: combination of obesity with low muscle mass (Stenholm et al., 2009)

Serotonin: a chemical that carries messages between nerve cells in the brain and throughout your body. Serotonin plays a key role in such body functions as mood, sleep, digestion, nausea, wound healing, bone health, blood clotting and sexual desire (The Cleveland Clinic, 2022).

SSRI: Selective serotonin reuptake inhibitors, the most commonly prescribed antidepressants. They can ease symptoms of moderate to severe depression, are relatively safe, and typically cause fewer side effects than other types of antidepressants do (The Mayo Clinic, 2019).

Stress (physiological): a state of threatened homeodynamic balance caused by a stressor (Agorastos & Chrousos, 2021)

Stressor: any intrinsic or extrinsic stimuli, either real or perceived, that cause a fight or flight response in an organism (Agorastos & Chrousos, 2021).

Thermoreceptors: specialized nerve cells that are able to detect differences in temperature (Study.com, 2015).

Tumor Necrosis Factor (TNF): a cytokine produced by macrophages, natural killer (NK) cells, and lymphocytes (Maloy & Hughes, 2013).

Up regulation: the process by which a cell increases its response to a substance or signal from outside the cell to carry out a specific function (National Cancer Institute).

Vasomotor symptoms: a form of temperature dysfunction that occurs due to hormonal changes during menopause (Deecher & Dorries, 2007).

References

Agorastos, A., & Chrousos, G. P. (2021, July 21). The neuroendocrinology of stress: the stress-related continuum of chronic disease development. Molecular Psychiatry, 27(1), 502-513. https://doi.org/10.1038/s41380-021-01224-9

American Cancer Society. (2019, December 27). Immune Checkpoint Inhibitors and Their Side Effects—Cancer Vaccines and Their Side Effects—Cytokines and Their Side Effects. American Cancer Society. Retrieved July 5, 2022, from https://www.cancer.org/treatment/treatments-and-side-effects/treatment-types/immunotherapy/cytokines.html

American Psychological Association. (2019, October 30). Mindfulness meditation: A research-proven way to reduce stress. American Psychological Association. Retrieved July 3, 2022, from https://www.apa.org/topics/mindfulness/meditation

Ana, R., García Rodríguez, L. A., Johansson, S., & Wallander, M.-A. (2003, Feb 25). Is hormone replacement therapy associated with an increased risk of irritable bowel syndrome? Maturitas: An international Journal of Midlife and Beyond, 44(2), 133-144. **https://doi.org/10.1016/S0378-5122(02)00321-3**

APA Div. 12 (Society of Clinical Psychology). (2017, July). What is Cognitive Behavioral Therapy? American Psychological Association. Retrieved July 2, 2022, from https://www.apa.org/ptsd-guideline/patients-and-families/cognitive-behavioral

Arthritis Foundation. (2021, Oct 15). Rheumatoid Arthritis: Causes, Symptoms, Treatments and More. Arthritis Foundation. Retrieved July 10, 2022, from https://www.arthritis.org/diseases/rheumatoid-arthritis

Banks, W. A., Kastin, A. J., & Gutierrez, E. G. (1996, Sept 26). Penetration of interleukin-6 across the murine blood-brain barrier. Neuroscience Letters, 179(1-2), 53-56. https://doi.org/10.1016/0304-3940(94)90933-4

Baxter, R. (n.d.). Types of muscle cells: Characteristics, location, roles. Kenhub. Retrieved July 9, 2022, from https://www.kenhub.com/en/library/anatomy/types-of-muscle-cells

Bonilla, C., Ness, A. R., Wills, A. K., Lawlor, D. A., Lewis, S. J., & Smith, G. D. (2014, Jun 12). Skin pigmentation, sun exposure and vitamin D levels in children of the Avon Longitudinal Study of Parents and Children. BMC public health, 14, 597. 10.1186/1471-2458-14-597

Boyce, B. F., Yao, Z., & Xing, L. (2010, Apr 19). Osteoclasts have Multiple Roles in Bone in Addition to Bone Resorption. Critical reviews in eukaryotic gene expression, 19(3), 171–180. 10.1615/critreveukargeneexpr.v19.i3.10

Brady, C. W. (2015, 7 Jul). Liver disease in menopause. World journal of gastroenterology, 21(25), 7613–7620. 10.3748/wjg.v21.i25.7613

Bremer, J. (1983, Oct 01). Carnitine--metabolism and functions. Physiological Reviews, 63(4), 1420-1480. https://doi.org/10.1152/physrev.1983.63.4.1420

Breuil, V., Ticchioni, M., Testa, J., Roux, C. H., Ferrari, P., Breittmayer, J. P., Albert-Sabonnadière, C., Durant, J., Perreti, F. D., Bernard, A., Euller-Ziegler, L., & Carle, G. F. (2009, October 30). Immune changes in post-menopausal osteoporosis: the Immunos study. Osteoporosis International, 21, 805–814. https://doi.org/10.1007/s00198-009-1018-7

Broekmans, F. J., Soules, M. R., & Fauser, B. C. (2009, Aug 30). Ovarian aging: mechanisms and clinical consequences. Endocrine reviews, 30(5), 465–493. 10.1210/er.2009-0006

Bromberger, J. T., Assmann, S. F., Avis, N. E., Schoken, M., Kravitz, H. M., & Cordal, A. (2003, August 15). Persistent mood symptoms in a multiethnic community cohort of pre- and perimenopausal women. American Journal of Epidemiology, 158(4), 347-356. https://doi.org/10.1016/j.psyneuen.2021.105128

Bryce, E. (2019, November 9). How Many Calories Can the Brain Burn by Thinking? Live Science. Retrieved July 8, 2022, from https://www.livescience.com/burn-calories-brain.html

Campbell, N. (2006). Biology Exploring Life (6th ed.). Pearson Prentice Hall.

Clausen, L. S., Abilgaard, A. B., Gersing, S. K., Stein, A., Lindorff-Larsen, K., & Hatmann-Petersen, R. (2019). Chapter Two - Protein stability and degradation in health and disease. Advances in Protein Chemistry and Structural Biology, 114, 61-83. https://doi.org/10.1016/bs.apcsb.2018.09.002

The Cleveland Clinic. (2022, March 18). Serotonin: What Is It, Function & Levels. Cleveland Clinic. Retrieved July 13, 2022, from https://my.clevelandclinic.org/health/articles/22572-serotonin

Columbia Neurosurgery. (n.d.). Cerebral Ischemia Diagnosis & Treatment - NYC | Columbia Neurosurgery in New York City. Columbia Neurosurgery. Retrieved July 10, 2022, from https://www.neurosurgery.columbia.edu/patient-care/conditions/cerebral-ischemia

Costello, R. B., Lentino, C. V., Boyd, C. C., O'Connell, M. L., Crawford, C. C., Sprengel, M. L., & Deuster, P. A. (2014, Nov 7). The effectiveness of melatonin for promoting healthy sleep: a rapid evidence assessment of the literature. Nutrition journal, 13, 106. 10.1186/1475-2891-13-106

Dabravolski, S. A., Nikiforov, N. G., Starodubova, A. V., Popkova, T. V., & Orekhov, A. N. (2021, Aug 16). The Role of Mitochondria-Derived Peptides in Cardiovascular Diseases and Their Potential as Therapeutic Targets. International journal of molecular sciences, 22(16), 8770. https://doi.org/10.3390/ijms22168770

Daneshzad, E., Keshavarz, S.-A., Qorbani, M., Larijani, B., & Azadbakht, L. (2020, Jun). Dietary total antioxidant capacity and its association with sleep, stress, anxiety, and depression score: A cross-sectional study among diabetic women. Clinical nutrition ESPEN, 37, 187–194. 10.1016/j.clnesp.2020.03.002

Deecher, D. C., & Dorries, K. (2007, Dec 12). Understanding the pathophysiology of vasomotor symptoms (hot flushes and night sweats) that occur in perimenopause, menopause, and postmenopause life stages. Archives of Women's Mental Health, 10(6), 247-57. https://doi.org/10.1007/s00737-007-0209-5

Deeks, A. A., & McCabe, M. P. (2004, April 17). Well-being and menopause: An investigation of purpose in life, self-acceptance, and social role in premenopausal, perimenopausal and postmenopausal women. Quality of Life Research, 13(2), 389–398. **https://doi.org/10.1023/B:QURE.0000018506.33706.05**

Dempsey, P. W., Vaidya, S. A., & Cheng, G. (2003, December). The Art of War: Innate and adaptive immune responses. Cellular and Molecular Life Sciences CMLS, 60, 2604–2621. Issue Date

Deng, F., Li, Y., & Zhao, J. (2019, Jan 15). The gut microbiome of healthy long-living people. Aging, 11(2), 289–290. https://doi.org/10.18632/aging.101771

de Wit, A. E., Giltay, E. J., de Boer, M. K., Nathan, M., Wiley, A., Crawford, S., & Joffe, H. (2021, April). Predictors of irritability symptoms in mildly depressed perimenopausal women. Psychoneuroendocrinology, 126. https://doi.org/10.1016/j.psyneuen.2021.105128

Dirckx, N., Moorer, M. C., Clemens, T. L., & Riddle, R. C. (2019, August 28). The role of osteoblasts in energy homeostasis. Nature Reviews Endocrinology, 15, pages651–665. https://doi.org/10.1038/s41574-019-0246-y

Dureshahwar, K., & Mohammad, W. (n.d.). Effects of Intermittent Fasting on Cognition and Neurodegeneration. Pakistan Journal of Neurological Sciences, 16(3), 34-37. https://ecommons.aku.edu/cgi/viewcontent.cgi?article=1536&context=pjns

Ebtekar, F., Davland, S., & Gheshlagh, R. G. (2018, Nov 1). The prevalence of metabolic syndrome in postmenopausal women: A systematic review and meta-analysis in Iran. Diabetes & metabolic syndrome, 12(6), 955–960. 10.1016/j.dsx.2018.06.002

Eldridge, L. (2022, February 22). Free Radicals: Definition, Cause, and Role in Cancer. Verywell Health. Retrieved July 7, 2022, from https://www.verywellhealth.com/information-about-free-radicals-2249103

Encyclopedia Britannica. (n.d.). adipose cell | Description, Types, & Function | Britannica. Encyclopedia Britannica. Retrieved July 6, 2022, from https://www.britannica.com/science/adipose-cell

Fasano, A. (2011, November 23). Leaky Gut and Autoimmune Diseases. Clinical Reviews in Allergy & Immunology, 42, 71-78. https://doi.org/10.1007/s12016-011-8291-x

Fink, G., Pfaff, D. W., & Levine, J. (Eds.). (2012). Handbook of Neuroendocrinology. Elsevier Science.

Freedman, R. R., & Suzanne, W. (1995). Altered Shivering Threshold in Postmenopausal Women with Hot Flashes. Menopause, 2(3), 163-168.

Frémont, L. (2000, January 14). Biological effects of resveratrol. Life Sciences, 66(8), 663-673. https://doi.org/10.1016/S0024-3205(99)00410-5

Galán, A. I., Palacios, E., Ruiz, F., Díez, A., Arji, M., Almar, M., Moreno, C., Calvo, J. I., Muñoz, M. E., Delgado, M. A., & Jiménez, R. (n.d.). Exercise, oxidative stress, and risk of cardiovascular disease in the elderly. Protective role of antioxidant functional foods. BioFactors, 27(1-4), 167–183. 10.1002/biof.5520270115.

Gameiro, C., & Romao, F. (2010, June 1). Changes in the immune system during menopause and aging. Frontiers in Bioscience, 2(4), 1299-1303. https://doi.org/10.2741/E190

Gilbert, N. (2022, January 27). When depression sneaks up on menopause. Knowable Magazine. Retrieved June 30, 2022, from https://knowablemagazine.org/article/mind/2022/when-depression-sneaks-menopause

Gold, E. B., Colvin, A., Avis, N., & Joyce Bromberger. (2011, October 10). Longitudinal Analysis of the Association Between Vasomotor Symptoms and Race/Ethnicity Across the Menopausal Transition: Study of Women's Health Across the Nation. American Journal of Public Health, 96, 1226-1235. https://doi.org/10.2105/AJPH.2005.066936

Golob, A. L., & Laya, M. B. (2015). Osteoporosis: Screening, Prevention and Management. Medical Clinics of North America, 99(3), 587-606. https://doi.org/10.1016/j.mcna.2015.01.010

Gray, D. A., & Woulfe, J. (2005, Feb 2). Lipofuscin and Aging: A Matter of Toxic Waste. SCIENCE OF AGING KNOWLEDGE ENVIRONMENT, 2005(5), re1. DOI: 10.1126/sageke.2005.5.re

Gruebner, O., Rapp, M. A., Adli, M., Kluge, U., Galea, S., & Heinz, A. (n.d.). Cities and Mental Health. Deutsches Arzteblatt international, 114(8), 121–127. https://doi.org/10.3238/arztebl.2017.0121

Guo, H., Callaway, J. B., & Ting, J. P.-Y. (2015, June 29). Inflammasomes: mechanism of action, role in disease, and therapeutics. Nature Medicine, 21, 677–687. https://doi.org/10.1038/nm.3893

Hamilton-Fairley, D., & Taylor, A. (2003, Sep 6). Anovulation. BMJ (Clinical research ed.), 327(7414), 546–549. https://doi.org/10.1136/bmj.327.7414.546

Hanauer, S.B., Campieri, M., Jewell, D.P., Rachmilewitz, D., Fiocchi, C., & Schölmerich, J. (Eds.). (2002). Inflammatory Bowel Disease: A Clinical Case Approach to Pathophysiology, Diagnosis, and Treatment. Springer Netherlands.

Haustein, C. H. (2019, Dec 15). Oxidation-reduction reaction. The Gale Encyclopedia of Science. Retrieved July 8, 2022, from https://go.gale.com/ps/i.do?p=SCIC&u=dc_demo&id=GALE|CV2644031629&v=2.1&it=r&sid=SCIC&asid=baa9fde9

Hayyan, M., Hashim, M. A., & AlNashef, I. M. (2016, Feb 15). Superoxide Ion: Generation and Chemical Implications. Chemical

Reviews, 116(5), 3029–3085. https://doi.org/10.1021/acs.chemrev.5b00407

He, S., Li, H., Yu, Z., Zhang, F., Liang, S., Liu, H., Chen, H., & Lu, M. (2021, Sep 28). The Gut Microbiome and Sex Hormone-Related Diseases. Frontiers in microbiology, 12(711137). 10.3389/fmicb.2021.711137

Hildreth, K. L., Ozemek, C., Kohrt, W. M., Blatchford, P. J., & Moreau, K. L. (2019, Sep 1). Vascular dysfunction across the stages of the menopause transition is associated with menopausal symptoms and quality of life. Menopause, 25(9), 1011–1019. 10.1097/GME.0000000000001112

Hou, M.-F., Ou-Yang, F., Li, C.-L., Chen, F.-M., Chuang, C.-H., Kan, J.-Y., Wu, C.-C., Shih, S.-L., Shaiu, J.-P., Kao, L.-C., Kao, C.-N., Lee, Y.-C., Moi, S.-H., Yeh, Y.-T., Cheng, C.-J., & Chiang, C.-P. (2021, October 27). Comprehensive profiles and diagnostic value of menopausal-specific gut microbiota in premenopausal breast cancer. Experimental and Molecular Medicine, 53, 1636–1646. https://doi.org/10.1038/s12276-021-00686-9

Iber, F. L., Murphy, P. A., & Connor, E. S. (1994, Jul 5). Age-related changes in the gastrointestinal system. Effects on drug therapy. Drugs & aging, 5(1), 34–48. 10.2165/00002512-199405010-00004

Jentsch, T. J., Stein, V., Weinreich, F., & Zdebik, A. A. (2002, Apr 1). Molecular Structure and Physiological Function of Chloride Channels. Physiological Reviews, 82(2). https://doi.org/10.1152/physrev.00029.2001

Jiang, B., Li, D., Larsen, L., & Sullivan, W. C. (2014, September 25). A Dose-Response Curve Describing the Relationship Between Urban Tree Cover Density and Self-Reported Stress Recovery. Environment and Behavior, 48(4), 607-629. https://doi.org/10.1177/0013916514552321

Johnell, O., & Kanis, J. A. (2006, Dec 17). An estimate of the worldwide prevalence and disability associated with osteoporotic fractures. Osteoporosis international: a journal established as result of cooperation between the European Foundation for Osteoporosis and the National Osteoporosis Foundation of the USA, 17(12), 1726–1733. 10.1007/s00198-006-0172-4

Johns Hopkins Medicine. (n.d.). Dysmenorrhea. Johns Hopkins Medicine. Retrieved July 6, 2022, from https://www.hopkinsmedicine.org/health/conditions-and-diseases/dysmenorrhea

Jung-Ha, K., Jee-Aee, I., & Duk-Chul, L. (2012, May). The relationship between leukocyte mitochondrial DNA contents and metabolic syndrome in postmenopausal women. The Journal of The North American Menopause Society, 19(5), 582-587. 10.1097/gme.0b013e31823a3e46

Kandasamy, M., Radhakrishnan1, R. K., Abirami, G. P. P., Roshan, S. A., Yesudhas, A., Balamuthu, K., Prahalathan, C., Shanmugaapriya, S., Moorthy, A., Essa, M. M., & Anusuyadevi, M. (2019, June 28). Possible Existence of the Hypothalamic-Pituitary-Hippocampal (HPH) Axis: A Reciprocal Relationship Between Hippocampal Specifc Neuroestradiol Synthesis and Neuroblastosis in Ageing Brains with Special Reference to Menopause and Neurocognitive Disorders. Neurochemical Research, 44, 1781–1795. **https://doi.org/10.1007/s11064-019-02833-1**

Kim, J.-H., Kwak, H.-B., Leewenburgh, C., & Lawler, J. M. (2008, April). Lifelong exercise and mild (8%) caloric restriction attenuate age-induced alterations in plantaris muscle morphology, oxidative stress, and IGF-1 in the Fischer-344 rat. Experimental Gerontology, 43(4), 317-329. https://doi.org/10.1016/j.exger.2007.12.012

Ko, Seong-Hee, & Kim, Hyun-Sook (2020, January 13). Menopause-Associated Lipid Metabolic Disorders and Foods Beneficial for Postmenopausal Women. Nutrients, Special Issue, "The Role of Diet in Menopause & Andropause) https://doi.org/10.3390/nu12010202

Kuhl, H. (2005). Pharmacology of estrogens and progestogens: influence of different routes of administration. Climateric, 8, 3–63. https://doi.org/10.1080/13697130500148875

Lahiri, S., Kim, H., Garcia-Perez, I., Maisha Reza, M., Martin, K. A., Kundu, P., Cox, L. M., Selkrig, J., Posma, J. M., Zhang, H., Pabmanabhan, P., Moret, C., Gulyás, B., Blaser, M. J., Auwerx, J., Holmes, E., Nicholson, J., Wahli, W., & Petterson, S. (2019, Jul 24). The gut microbiota influences skeletal muscle mass and function in mice. Science translational medicine, 11(502). 10.1126/scitranslmed.aan5662

Lanza, I. R., Zabielski, P., Klaus, K. A., Morse, D. M., Heppelmann, C. J., Bergen III, H.R., Dasari, S., Walrand, S., Short, K. R., Johnson, M. L., Robinson, M. M., Schimke, J. M., Jakaitis, D. R., Asmann, Y. W., Sun, Z., & Nair, K. S. (2012, Dec 5). Chronic Caloric Restriction Preserves Mitochondrial Function in Senescence Without Increasing Mitochondrial Biogenesis. Cell metabolism, 16(6), 777–788. https://doi.org/10.1016/j.cmet.2012.11.003

Li, S., Mao, Y., Zhou, F., Yang, H., Shi, Q., & Meng, B. (2020, August). Gut Microbiome and Osteoporosis, Bone Joint Res, 9(8), 524-530. https://doi.org/10.1302/2046-3758.98.BJR-2020-0089.R1

Lian, J., Yue, Y., Yu, W., & Zhang, Y. (2020, September 23). Immunosenescence: a key player in cancer development. Journal of Hematology & Oncology, 13, 151. https://doi.org/10.1186/s13045-020-00986-z

Liu, T., Li, N., Yan, Y., Liu, Y., Xiong, K., Liu, Y., Xia, Q., Zhang, H., & Liu, Z. (2020, Mar). Recent advances in the anti-aging effects of phytoestrogens on collagen, water content, and oxidative stress. Phytotherapy research: PTR, 34(3), 435–447. https://doi.org/10.1002/ptr.6538

Lopaschuk, G. D., Ussher, J. R., Folmes, C. D.L., Jaswal, J. S., & Stanley, W. C. (2010, Jan 1). Myocardial Fatty Acid Metabolism in Health and Disease. Physiological Reviews, 90(1), 207-258. https://doi.org/10.1152/physrev.00015.2009

Lozano, R., Nahavi, M., Foreman, K., Lim, S., Shibuya, K., Aboyans, V., Abraham, J., Adair, T., Aggarwal, R., Ahn, S. Y., Alvarado, M.,

Anderson, R., & Anderson, L. M. (2012, Dec 15). Global and regional mortality from 235 causes of death for 20 age groups in 1990 and 2010: a systematic analysis for the Global Burden of Disease Study 2010. Lancet, 380(9859), 2095–2128. 10.1016/S0140-6736(12)61728-0

Maki, P. M., Kornstein, S. G., Joffe, H., Bromberger, J. T., Freeman, E. W., Athappilly, G., Bobo, W. V., Rubin, L. H., Cohen, L. S., & Soares, C. N. (2019, Feb 14). Guidelines for the Evaluation and Treatment of Perimenopausal Depression: Summary and Recommendations. Journal of Women's Health, 28(2), 117-134. https://doi.org/10.1089/jwh.2018.27099.mensocrec

Maloy, S., & Hughes, K. (Eds.). (2013). Brenner's Encyclopedia of Genetics. Elsevier Science.

Marks, A. D., Peet, A., & Lieberman, M. (2013). Marks' Basic Medical Biochemistry: A Clinical Approach (M. Lieberman & A. D. Marks, Eds.). Wolter Kluwer Health/Lippincott Williams & Wilkins.

Marotta, F., Marcellino, M., Catanzaro, R., Campiotti, A., Lorenzetti, A., Cervi, J., & Barbagallo, M. (2020, January 10). Mitochondrial and Redox Dysfunction in Post-Menopause as Risk Factor of Neurodegenerative Disease: A Pilot Study Testing the Role of a Validated Japanese Functional Food. Journal of Biological Regulators & Homeostatic Agents, 34(1), 47-57. 10.23812/19-315-A

Martin, J. H. (2003). Neuroanatomy: Text and Atlas. McGraw-Hill.

Martins, E. (2014, Jan 10). The growing use of herbal medicines: issues relating to adverse reactions and challenges in monitoring safety. Frontiers in Pharmacology, 4(177). 10.3389/fphar.2013.00177

Marzetti, E., Lees, H. A., Wohlgemuth, S. E., & Leeuwenburgh, C. (2009, Feb). Sarcopenia of aging: underlying cellular mechanisms and protection by calorie restriction. Biofactors, 35(1), 28-35. 10.1002/biof.5

The Mayo Clinic. (2019, Sept 17). Selective serotonin reuptake inhibitors (SSRIs). Mayo Clinic. Retrieved July 2, 2022, from https://www.mayoclinic.org/diseases-conditions/depression/in-depth/ssris/art-20044825

Mayo Clinic. (2021, February 18). Amenorrhea - Symptoms and causes. Mayo Clinic. Retrieved July 10, 2022, from https://www.mayoclinic.org/diseases-conditions/amenorrhea/symptoms-causes/syc-20369299

The Mayo Clinic. (2021, December 1). Irritable bowel syndrome - Symptoms and causes. Mayo Clinic. Retrieved July 5, 2022, from https://www.mayoclinic.org/diseases-conditions/irritable-bowel-syndrome/symptoms-causes/syc-20360016

McAuley, M. T., Kenny, R. A., Kirkwood, T. B., Wilkinson, D. J., Jones, J. J., & Miller, V. M. (2009, MAr 25). A mathematical model of aging-related and cortisol induced hippocampal dysfunction. BMC Neuroscience, 10(26). https://doi.org/10.1186/1471-2202-10-26

McQueen, C. (Ed.). (2010). Comprehensive Toxicology (Second ed.). Elsevier Science. https://www.elsevier.com/books/comprehensive-toxicology/9780080468846

Merriam-Webster. ((n.d.)). Homeostasis. Merriam-Webster. https://www.merriam-webster.com/dictionary/homeostasis

Merry, T. L., Chan, A., Woodhead, J. S.T., Reynolds, J. C., Kumagai, H., & Kim, S.-J. (2020, Sept 20). Mitochondrial-derived peptides in energy metabolism. American Journal of Physiology-Endocrinology and Metabolism, 319(4). https://doi.org/10.1152/ajpendo.00249.2020

Min, J., Jo, H., Chung, Y.-J., Song, J. Y., Kim, M. J., & Kim, M.-R. (2021, Dec 14). Vitamin D and the Immune System in Menopause: A Review. Journal of menopausal medicine, 27(3), 109–114. 10.6118/jmm.21011

Mitchell, L. (2020, July 30). Your gut bacteria's superpower: Butyrate | Microba. Microba Insight. Retrieved July 5, 2022, from https://insight.microba.com/blog/your-gut-bacterias-superpower-butyrate/

Mizushima, N., & Komatsu, M. (2011, Nov 11). Autophagy: Renovation of Cells and Tissues. Cellpress, 147(4), 728-741. https://doi.org/10.1016/j.cell.2011.10.026

Montoya-Estrada, A., Veruete-Bedolla, D. B., Romo-Yañez, J., Ortiz-Luna, G. F., Arellano-Eguiluz, A., Nájera, N., Ceballos, G., Nieto-Velázquez, N. G., Ramos-Valencia, M. A., Cariño-Mancilla, N., & Valdez-Rodríguez, N. L. (2022, Jun 01). Markers of oxidative stress in postmenopausal women with metabolic syndrome. Journal of Obstetrics and Gynaecology. https://doi.org/10.1080/01443615.2022.2062223

Nathan, M. D., Wiley, A., Mahon, P. B., Camuso, J., Sullivan, K., McCormick, K., Srivastava, A., Kim, A., Newhouse, P., & Joffe, H. (2021, April). Hypothalamic-pituitary-adrenal axis, subjective, and thermal stress responses in midlife women with vasomotor symptoms. Menopause, 28(4), 439-443. 10.1097/GME.0000000000001703

National Cancer Institute. (n.d.). Definition of apoptosis - NCI Dictionary of Cancer Terms - NCI. National Cancer Institute. Retrieved July 20, 2022, from https://www.cancer.gov/publications/dictionaries/cancer-terms/def/apoptosis

National Cancer Institute. (n.d.). Definition of gastrointestinal tract - NCI Dictionary of Cancer Terms - NCI. National Cancer Institute. Retrieved July 4, 2022, from https://www.cancer.gov/publications/dictionaries/cancer-terms/def/gastrointestinal-tract

National Cancer Institute. (n.d.). Definition of nocebo effect - NCI Dictionary of Cancer Terms - NCI. National Cancer Institute. Retrieved July 14, 2022, from https://www.cancer.gov/publications/dictionaries/cancer-terms/def/nocebo-effect

National Cancer Institute. (n.d.). Definition of upregulation - NCI Dictionary of Cancer Terms - NCI. National Cancer Institute. Retrieved July 15, 2022, from https://www.cancer.gov/publications/dictionaries/cancer-terms/def/upregulation

National Cancer Institute. (n.d.). Definition of white blood cell - NCI Dictionary of Cancer Terms - NCI. National Cancer Institute. Retrieved July 2, 2022, from https://www.cancer.gov/publications/dictionaries/cancer-terms/def/white-blood-cell

National Center for Chronic Disease Prevention and Health Promotion. (2021, July 19). Coronary Artery Disease | cdc.gov. Centers for Disease Control and Prevention. Retrieved July 4, 2022, from https://www.cdc.gov/heartdisease/coronary_ad.htm

National Health Service. (2019). Metabolic syndrome. NHS. Retrieved July 8, 2022, from https://www.nhs.uk/conditions/metabolic-syndrome/#

National Heart, Lung, and Blood Institute. (2022, March 24). Atherosclerosis - What Is Atherosclerosis? NHLBI. Retrieved July 12, 2022, from https://www.nhlbi.nih.gov/health/atherosclerosis#

National Institute of Diabetes and Digestive and Kidney Diseases. (2018). Gonadotropins. National Institute of Diabetes and Digestive and Kidney Diseases. https://pubmed.ncbi.nlm.nih.gov/31644163/#

National Institute of Environmental Health Sciences. (2022, April 05). Microbiome. National Institute of Environmental Health Sciences. Retrieved July 4, 2022, from https://www.niehs.nih.gov/health/topics/science/microbiome/index.cfm

National Institute of Neurological Disorders and Stroke. (2022, April 1). Brain Basics: Understanding Sleep | National Institute of Neurological Disorders and Stroke. National Institute of Neurological Disorders and Stroke. Retrieved June 30, 2022, from https://www.ninds.nih.gov/health-information/patient-caregiver-education/brain-basics-understanding-sleep

Nguyen, J. K., & Thurston, R. C. (2020, December 10). Association of Childhood Trauma Exposure with Inflammatory Biomarkers Among Midlife Women. Journal of Women's Health, 29(12), 1540-1546. https://doi.org/10.1089/jwh.2019.7779

Oliveira, P. J., Carvalho, R. A., Portincasa, P., Bonfrate, L., & Sardao, V. A. (2012, Feb 01). Fatty Acid Oxidation and Cardiovascular Risk during Menopause: A Mitochondrial Connection? Journal of Lipids, 2012, 12. https://doi.org/10.1155/2012/365798

Pandey, K. B., & Ibrahim Rizvi, S. (2009, Nov-Dec). Plant polyphenols as dietary antioxidants in human health and disease. Oxidative medicine and cellular longevity, 2(5), 270–278. https://doi.org/10.4161/oxim.2.5.9498

Pappan, N., & Rehman, A. (2022). Dyslipidemia. StatPearls Publishing.

Paulus, M. P. (2015, Dec 10). Neural Basis of Mindfulness Interventions that Moderate the Impact of Stress on the Brain. Neuropsychopharmacology: official publication of the American College of Neuropsychopharmacology, 41(1), 373. 10.1038/npp.2015.239

Pereira, G. A., da Silva, A., Hermsdorff, H. H. M., & Boroni Moreira, A. P. (2021, September 27). Association of dietary total antioxidant capacity with depression, anxiety, and sleep disorders: A systematic review of observational studies. Journal of Clinical and Translational Research, 7(5), 631-640. https://pubmed.ncbi.nlm.nih.gov/34778593/

Petrine, J. C.P., & Del Bianco-Borges, B. (2020, August 11). The influence of phytoestrogens on different physiological and pathological processes: An overview. Phytotherapy Research, 35(1), 180-197. https://doi.org/10.1002/ptr.6816

Pizzino, G., Irrera, N., Cucinotta, M., Pallio, G., Mannino, F., Arcoraci, V., Squadrito, F., Altavilla, D., & Bitto, A. (2017). Oxidative Stress: Harms and Benefits for Human Health. Oxidative medicine and cellular longevity. 10.1155/2017/8416763

Pramyothin, P., & Holick, M. F. (2012, Mar). Vitamin D supplementation: guidelines and evidence for subclinical deficiency. Current opinion in gastroenterology, 28(2), 139–150. https://doi.org/10.1097/MOG.0b013e32835004dc

Robertson, S. (2018, August 23). What are Amyloid Plaques? News-Medical.net. Retrieved July 10, 2022, from https://www.news-medical.net/health/What-are-Amyloid-Plaques.aspx

Roh, J. S., & Sohn, D. H. (2018, Aug 13). Damage-Associated Molecular Patterns in Inflammatory Diseases. Immune Network, 18(4), e27. https://doi.org/10.4110/in.2018.18.e27

Saldana, J. I. (n.d.). Macrophages | British Society for Immunology. British Society for Immunology |. Retrieved July 11, 2022, from https://www.immunology.org/public-information/bitesized-immunology/cells/macrophages

Sampson, J. N., Falk, R. T., Schairer, C., Moore, S. C., Fuhrman, B. J., Dallal, C. M., Bauer, D. C., Dorgan, J. F., Shu, X.-O., Zheng, W., Brinton, L. A., Gail, M. H., Ziegler, R. G., Xu, X., Hoover, R. N., & Gierach, G. L. (2017, Feb). Association of Estrogen Metabolism with Breast Cancer Risk in Different Cohorts of Postmenopausal Women. American Association for Cancer Research, 77(4), 918–925. https://doi.org/10.1158/0008-5472.CAN-16-1717

Schaffler, M. B., Cheung, W.-Y., Majeska, R., & Kennedy, O. (2015, Jan 1). Osteocytes: Master Orchestrators of Bone. Calcified tissue international, 94(1), 5-24. https://doi.org/10.1007/s00223-013-9790-y

Seeley, T. D. (1995). The wisdom of the hive: the social physiology of honeybee colonies. Harvard University Press.

Seib, C., Whiteside, E., Lee, K., Humphreys, J., Dao Tran, T. H., Chopin, L., & Anderson, D. (2014, Feb). Stress, lifestyle, and quality of life in midlife and older Australian women: results from the Stress and the Health of Women Study. Women's Health Issues, 24(1), 43-52. https://doi.org/10.1016/j.whi.2013.11.004

Shea, A. K., Frey, B. N., Gervais, N., Lopez, A., & Minuzzi, L. (2021, May 05). Depression in midlife women attending a menopause clinic is associated with a history of childhood maltreatment. Climateric, 25(2), 203-207. https://doi.org/10.1080/13697137.2021.1915270

Shieh, A., Epeldegui, M., Karlamangla, A., & Greendale, G. A. (2020, Jan 30). Gut permeability, inflammation, and bone density across the menopause transition. JCI insight, 5(2). https://doi.org/10.1172/jci.insight.134092

Shin, B. K., Kang, S., & Kim, d. S. (2018, Jan 7). Intermittent fasting protects against the deterioration of cognitive function, energy metabolism and dyslipidemia in Alzheimer's disease-induced estrogen deficient rats. Experimental Biology and Medicine, 243(4), 334-343. 10.1177/1535370217751610

Shriver, E. K. (2013, June 28). Menopause: Overview. National Institute of Child Health and Human Development. https://web.archive.org/web/20150402111845/http://www.nichd.nih.gov/health/topics/menopause/Pages/default.aspx

Sievert, L. L., Jaff, N., & Woods, N. F. (2016, March 16). Stress and midlife women's health. Women's Midlife Health, 4. https://doi.org/10.1186/s40695-018-0034-1

Singh, I. (2011). Textbook of Anatomy: Volume 3: Head and Neck, Central Nervous System. Jaypee Brothers Medical Publishers Pvt. Limited.

Society for Endocrinology. (2019, Jan). Cortisol. You and Your Hormones. Retrieved July 1, 2022, from https://www.yourhormones.info/hormones/cortisol/

Sporns, O. (2014, May 20). Connectome. Scholarpedia. Retrieved July 15, 2022, from http://www.scholarpedia.org/article/Connectome

Stenholm, S., Harris, T. B., Rantanen, T., Visser, M., Kritchevsky, S. B., & Ferrucci, L. (2009, Jan 30). Sarcopenic obesity - definition, etiology, and consequences. Curr Opin Clin Nutr Metab Care, 11(6), 693-700. 10.1097/MCO.0b013e328312c37d

Study.com. (2015, October 16). Thermoreceptors: Definition & Function. Study.com. Retrieved July 13, 2022, from https://study.com/academy/lesson/thermoreceptors-definition-function-quiz.html

Tansey, E. A., & Johnson, C. D. (2015, Sep 01). Recent advances in thermoregulation. Advances in Physiology Education, 39(3), 139-148. https://doi.org/10.1152/advan.00126.2014

Tolfrey, K. (2010). American Heart Association Guidelines for Preventing Heart Disease in Women: 2007 Update. The Physician and Sportsmedicine, 38(1), 162-164. 10.3810/psm.2010.04.1774

Turnbaugh, P. J., Hamady, M., Yatsunenko, T., Cantarel, B. L., Duncan, A., Ley, R. E., Sogin, M. L., Jones, W. J., Roe, B. A., Affourtit, J. P., Egholm, M., Henrissat, B., Heath, A. C., Knight, R., & Gordon, J. I. (2008, Nov 30). A core gut microbiome in obese and lean twins. Nature, 457(7228), 480–484. https://doi.org/10.1038/nature07540

Uribe-Querol, E., & Rosales, C. (2020, June 02). Phagocytosis: Our Current Understanding of a Universal Biological Process. Frontiers in Immunology, (02), Jun. https://doi.org/10.3389/fimmu.2020.01066

van Driel, C., de Bock, G., Schroevers, M., & Mourits, M. (2018, September 17). Mindfulness-based stress reduction for menopausal symptoms after risk-reducing salpingo-oophorectomy (PURSUE study): a randomized controlled trial. BJOG: An International Journal of Obstetrics & Gynecology, 126, 402-411. https://doi.org/10.1111/1471-0528.15471

Vanuytsel, T., Tack, J., & Farre, R. (2021, August 26). The Role of Intestinal Permeability in Gastrointestinal Disorders and Current Methods of Evaluation. Frontiers in Nutrition, 8. https://doi.org/10.3389/fnut.2021.717925

Vazquez, L. (2016, June 9). Scientists Now Know How Many Trees You Need to See to Relax. Big Think. Retrieved July 15, 2022, from https://bigthink.com/surprising-science/scientists-now-know-how-many-trees-you-need-to-see-to-relax/

Veloso, H. G. (n.d.). FODMAP Diet: What You Need to Know. Johns Hopkins Medicine. Retrieved July 5, 2022, from https://www.hopkinsmedicine.org/health/wellness-and-prevention/fodmap-diet-what-you-need-to-know

Verkhatsky, A., & Nedergaard, M. (2017, Dec 12). Physiology of Astroglia. Physiological Reviews, 98(1), 239-389. https://doi.org/10.1152/physrev.00042.2016

Vigna, J., Tontonoz, M., Shuster, M., & Sinha, G. (2014). Scientific American Biology for a Changing World with Core Physiology. W. H. Freeman.

Vincent, J., & Inassi, J. (2020, March 2). Comparison of oxidative stress between premenopausal and postmenopausal women. National Journal of Physiology, Pharmacy and Pharmacology, 10(5), 359-362.

Voss, P., Thomas, M. E., Cisneros-Franco, J. M., & de Villers-Sidani, '. (2017, October 04). Dynamic Brains and the Changing Rules of Neuroplasticity: Implications for Learning and Recovery. Frontiers in Psychology. https://doi.org/10.3389/fpsyg.2017.01657

Walsh, M. C., Kim, N., Kadono, Y., Rho, J., Lee, S. Y., Lorenzo, J., & Choi, Y. (2006, April 23). OSTEOIMMUNOLOGY: Interplay Between the Immune System and Bone Metabolism. Annual Review of Immunology, 24, 33-63. https://doi.org/10.1146/annurev.immunol.24.021605.090646

Walston, J. D. (2012, Nov). Sarcopenia in older adults. Current opinion in rheumatology, 24(6), 623–627. 10.1097/BOR.0b013e328358d59b

Wan-Qiang, L., Xu, L., Hui, S., Hui-Min, L., Xiang, Q., Bo-Yang, L., Wen-Di, S., Chang-Li, G., Feng-Ye, L., Jie, S., Hong-Mei, X., & Hong-Wen, D. (2021, September 01). Human gut microbiome impacts skeletal muscle mass via gut microbial synthesis of the short-chain fatty acid butyrate among healthy menopausal women. Journal of Cachexia, Sarcopenia and Muscle, 12(6), 1860-1870. https://doi.org/10.1002/jcsm.12788

White, Y. A. R., Woods, D. C., Takai, Y., Ishidara, O., Seki, H., & Tilly, J. L. (2012). Oocyte formation by mitotically active germ cells purified from ovaries of reproductive-age women. Nature Medicine, 18, 413–421. https://doi.org/10.1038/nm.2669

Xiang, D., Liu, Y., Zhou, S., Zhou, E., & Wang, Y. (2021, Jun 29). Protective Effects of Estrogen on Cardiovascular Disease Mediated by Oxidative Stress. Oxidative Medicine and Cellular Longevity, 2021. https://doi.org/10.1155/2021/5523516

Xiong, G. L., & Doraiswamy, P. M. (2009, August 28). Does Meditation Enhance Cognition and Brain Plasticity? Longevity, Regeneration, and Optimal Health Integrating Eastern and Western Perspectives, 1172(1), 63-69. 10.1007/s11064-019-02833-1

Yang, P.-L., Heitkemper, M. M., & Kamp, K. J. (2021, May 31). Irritable bowel syndrome in midlife women: a narrative review. Women's Midlife Health, 7(4). https://doi.org/10.1186/s40695-021-00064-5

Yashin, A., Yashin, Y., Wang, J. Y., & Nemzer, B. (2013, Dec 2). Antioxidant and Antiradical Activity of Coffee. Antioxidants (Basel, Switzerland), 2(4), 30–245. 10.3390/antiox2040230

Yihua, L., Yun, J., & Dongshen, Z. (2017, Mar 17). Coronary Artery Disease in Premenopausal and Postmenopausal Women. International Heart Journal, 58(2), 174-179. 10.1536/ihj.16-095

Yildiz, F. (Ed.). (2006). Phytoestrogens In Functional Foods. Taylor & Francis.

Yong, C. S., Kream, B. E., & Raisz, L. G. (1984, February 1). Cortisol Decreases Bone Formation by Inhibiting Periosteal Cell Proliferation. Endocrinology, 114(2), 477–480. https://doi.org/10.1210/endo-114-2-477

Zhao, H., Chen, J., Li, X., Sun, Q., Qin, P., & Wang, Q. (2019, July 05). Compositional and functional features of the female premenopausal and postmenopausal gut microbiota. FEBS Letters, 593(18), 2655-2664. https://doi.org/10.1002/1873-3468.13527